Wise, witty and wonderful. A must-read!

As the editor of a parenting website, I receive countless e-mails from women who are completely overwhelmed by all the books, research and well-intentioned advice given to pregnant moms. It's truly information overload.

That's what makes *A Simple Guide* such a refreshing read—it has everything new moms need to know, and none of the fluff. From managing pregnancy mood swings to tips for returning to work, Ivana shares practical advice in a way that's sure to inspire confidence. Wise, witty and wonderful—this book is a must-read for any mom-to-be!

~Megan Sayers, Managing Editor, Modern Mom

A valuable resource

A great comprehensive guide for pregnancy and baby's first year. This book does an excellent job of addressing the many questions a new mom may have during an uncertain and overwhelming time. The nutritional guidelines make it easy for any woman to adapt a healthier diet and lifestyle both for herself and baby. Filled with the most up-to-date information from vaccination schedules to monthly milestones, *A Simple Guide* is a valuable resource for any new mother or mother-to-be.

~Dr. Bess Raker, pediatrician
and co-founder of Beverly Hills Pediatrics

Healthy eats and fitness were an important part of my own pregnancy. I'm a Gourmet Mama myself and loved the delicious, nutritious recipes.

~Chef Lory Weissenberg-Abascal, co-host of
TV's *Utilísima,* and mother of two

If you are going to buy one book during your pregnancy, this is the one! *A Simple Guide* is the most fun book I have read about pregnancy and early motherhood! I have four kids and I wish I'd had it for all of my pregnancies. The advice makes you feel confident and the Quick & Easy tips are lifesavers.

~Jennifer Underwood, family CEO, mother of four

Step-by-step practical advice that builds confidence and brings results. Believe me, you will use this book over and over during your pregnancy and baby's first year.

~Melissa Miller, project manager, mother of two

Finally, a smart and funny book about pregnancy and new motherhood that covers all the essentials without weighing you down.

~Victoria O'Toole, bestselling children's author
of *Molly Moccasins,* and mother of twins

You're pregnant, tired, and overwhelmed. Info overload is not what you're after. *A Simple Guide* gives new moms what they need: expert advice, easy to understand and put into practice. All the basics covered in one convenient book.

~Jordan Roter, author of *Girl in Development,* mother of two

The Modern Princess:
A Simple Guide to Pregnancy
& Baby's First Year

The Modern Princess:
A Simple Guide to Pregnancy
& Baby's First Year

Princess Ivana Pignatelli Aragona Cortes
Magdalene Smith
Marisa Smith

DON'T SWEAT IT MEDIA, INC.

Don't Sweat It Media, Inc.

First Edition: April 2013

Acting Consultant Bess Raker M.D., F.A.A.P., Beverly Hills Pediatrics

Illustrations by Rima Hawkes

Jacket Photograph by Marisa Smith

Printed in the United States of America

Library of Congress Control No. 2013933333

ISBN-13: 978-0-9888712-0-5
epub ISBN: 978-0-9888712-1-2

NOTE TO READERS

This publication contains the ideas and opinions of its authors. It is intended to provide helpful and informative material on the subjects addressed in the publication. It is sold with the understanding that the authors and publisher are not engaged in rendering medical, health, or any other kind of personal professional services in the book. The reader should consult her or his medical, health, or other competent professional before adopting any of the suggestions in this book or drawing inferences from it.

The authors and publisher specifically disclaim all responsibility for any liability, loss, or risk, personal or otherwise, which is incurred as a consequence, directly or indirectly, of the use and application of any of the contents of this book.

This book identifies product names and services known to be trademarks, registered trademarks, or service marks of their respective holders. They are used throughout this book in an editorial fashion only. Use of a term in this book should not be regarded as affecting the validity of any trademark, registered trademark, or service mark. The Modern Princess/Princess Ivana is not associated with any product or vendor mentioned in this book.

Table of Contents

This book is dedicated to Alessio and Sienna—
thank you for inspiring me to be a better person and mommy,
and to my husband Adriano—thank you for all your love and support.

Acknowledgements

Special thanks to Jennifer, Missy, Dante, Martie, June, Tammy, Peggy, Gabby, Jill, Carolina, and all my girlfriends and mom friends for being part of this book by sharing your stories. With gratitude to Jordan Roter, Dottie DeHart, Heather Prestwood, Bess Raker, Kate Lee, Emma Sweeney, Elena Castillo, Jessica Beranek, and Megan Sayers—you have helped me in more ways than you know.

Above all, thank you to my family for giving me such inspiration and love throughout the years: Adriano, Alessio, Sienna, Papa (Joe Smith), Mommy (Magdalene Smith), Marisa Smith, Michael Smith, Nicolo Pignatelli, Susan Pignatelli, Tanja Pignatelli, Ascanio Pignatelli, Mama Lane, Aunt Cathy, Uncle Rand, & Auntie Lisanne.

Introduction

As a new parent who had spent most of my life attending to my career, the only thing I knew was that I *didn't* know when it came to babies and motherhood. Choices are a good thing, but I was overwhelmed by the tidal wave of information, education, baby products, medical research, do's and don'ts that seemed to change from article to article, book to book. Yes, I'm a real princess (we'll get to that later), but I'm also an Excel freak; a researcher and digital strategy consultant who depends on my beloved spreadsheets to make sense of a world that is ever-changing with new information even as I write this.

When I was four months pregnant with my first child, I put my research talents to work, scouring the Internet to get ideas on baby essentials for the first year. I was slammed by hundreds of products, ads posing as informative articles, and companies rolling out their wares in a dizzying array. Nearly every product made superlative claims. One guaranteed happiness. Another offered my baby a higher IQ, better muscle coordination and "a more secure self image." The bouncy walker claimed it could not only increase my baby's strength, but help my "little one on the path to bilingualism!"

How could I know who to believe, where to even begin? There are literally millions of choices for parents today. Thousands of toys, cribs, teething products, books on infancy and parenting. Google "tips on breastfeeding" and you get 18,600,000 results. One thing new mothers don't have is time to wade through the often conflicting mass of information, or the money to try every product that claims it is the best.

And so began my quest for the absolute essentials. The result is *A Simple Guide to Pregnancy & Baby's First Year*, a fun and easy-to-use reference that covers the most important aspects of pregnancy and your baby's first year. It is designed for busy moms, to help you smoothly adjust to the new life in your life, including budget-wise tips on baby basics. Keep it by your bed or in the nursery as a quick reference when questions arise on breastfeeding, eating and sleep schedules, and general developmental milestones.

I am a princess, but I'm just like you. I came from a regular family and we had to save and think about how to spend our money. My parents used to joke: "Here's a quarter—go buy yourself something special." The funny thing was, as a kid I often found "something special" that gave me pleasure and satisfaction, even on my shoestring allowance. So call me frugal, thrifty, a happy bargain hunter—the opposite of what you may think a princess might be. I know the value of how to live well, no matter how large or small your budget.

Being a princess has given me access to expertise—the best doctors and information, and enough resources to spare no cost when it comes to my babies' well-being. But the most important choices you will make as a parent have little to do with money, and everything to do with educating yourself, trusting your instincts, and paying attention to your child's signals.

This book is a combination of my personal experiences during pregnancy and new motherhood; best practices from friends, family, and national mothers' groups; and extensive research on parenting, health and child development.

I hope the practical advice and collective wisdom contained in this simple guide will contribute to your family's health and well-being for years to come!

Ciao!

Princess Ivana

About the Authors

Princess Ivana Maria Pignatelli Aragona Cortes is a modern Cinderella married to an Italian prince. Their 2 fabulous kids (ages two and three years) are the latest additions to a 1000-year lineage that includes kings of Sicily and Spain, Catherine of Aragon, a pope and a saint. Ivana is wild about kids and motherhood. For twenty years, she has worked with children—from designing learning toys to tutoring homeless kids. For Ivana, life is more about attitude than money. She came from modest means and met her Prince Charming while on scholarship at Pepperdine. She has a Masters in Education and is a digital strategy consultant. She is currently a popular featured blogger on Modern Mom. For more on Ivana, go to www.princessivana.com.

Magdalene Smith (Ivana's mom) received her MFA in Writing from Vermont College. She is the recipient of the University of New Mexico's Resident Writer's Award, two Wurlitzer Foundation fellowships, a Ludwig Vogelstein Foundation grant, and a Martin Foundation Creative Arts grant. Her work has been published in the U.S. and abroad.

Marisa Smith (Ivana's sister) has over fifteen years experience in fashion. A style consultant to some of the wealthiest women in the country, Marisa's expert sense of fashion made her one of Neiman Marcus' top Armani specialists. On a regular basis, the company flew her to Milan and New York to do multimillion-dollar buys for the Giorgio Armani boutique.

Illustrator: Rima Hawkes specializes in web design, graphic design and illustration. With over a decade of experience, she has worked for major high-end cosmetic companies with a passion for lifestyle, health, music, beauty, and fashion. Rima has dreamed of illustrating children's books since childhood. She has known Ivana and Marisa since they were all kids. A dear friend and close member of The Modern Princess team, Rima illustrates all the Princess Ivana blogs. Currently based in NYC, she holds a BFA in Graphic Design and an AA degree in Fine Art. www.rimahawkes.com

Acting Consultant: Bess Raker, M.D., F.A.A.P., is a board certified pediatrician and co-founder of Beverly Hills Pediatrics. Dr. Raker is committed to educating parents about how to raise healthy and happy children. She did her pediatric training at Children's Hospital Los Angeles and is currently affiliated with Cedars-Sinai Medical Center, ranked #1 in the Los Angeles Metropolitan Area in Maternity (Obstetrics) in 2012, and named one of America's best hospitals by *U.S. News & World Report* (2012-13).

The Modern Princess:
A Simple Guide to Pregnancy
& Baby's First Year

Chapter 1

Me? A Princess?

What little girl hasn't dreamed of being a princess? But princess is a loaded word, conjuring an impossible mix of fantasy, magic and romance. In fairytales, it is the end-all, be-all. The story of Cinderella ends with her becoming a princess. The happily-ever-after is never explained. Only that she has a prince, a castle, and enough money to do anything she wants. And then? We grow up and set out in search of our own happy-ever-afters.

A real-life Cinderella was ~~the~~ last thing on my mind as I applied for a scholarship to Pepperdine University when I was twenty-one. I wanted to be a business woman. International business. Entrepreneur, lawyer, something like that—where I would be my own woman. I came from modest means. I had been working since I was fourteen and understood the golden key to my dreams was an education, not Prince Charming.

So how did I become a princess?

First off, I got the scholarship to Pepperdine. I was a business major, honor student, double timing it as a Residential Advisor for my dorm, and First-Aid Responder for the volleyball team to offset college costs. Dream big, work hard—that's what my parents taught me.

When I met my future husband, I didn't know he was a prince. We met in a nightclub, introduced by mutual friends. Adriano had recently graduated from Pepperdine with his degree in International Studies. He was a charming Italian, good looking too, but I was at the midpoint of a promise to myself: no dating for six months. I had gone solo successfully for three. I wanted to get settled into my new life, and I wanted to get to know me. When Adriano offered me a drink, I showed him my glass and said, "I already have one." Maybe he liked my lack of interest in him. That night he secretly told his friend he was going to marry me, and I secretly decided six months was a long time to be alone.

In the early stages of dating, Adriano tried several times to tell me about his family. He wouldn't quite say what they did. He would start to talk about them, then stop abruptly, flustered. Sometimes he would ask me: "You know about my family, don't you?"

Okay, I'm not *that* old, but these were the days before Google and Facebook. The idea of looking somebody up and knowing his whole history in a few seconds just didn't exist. I didn't know a thing about Adriano's family, except that he was born in Rome and his family roots were in Naples. I figured they must be in the Mafia. Why else would Adriano act so weird? By then I was in falling in love with him, so crazy in love it almost didn't matter if there was a godfather or two in the closet.

Four months into our relationship, Adriano told me that he was a prince. I thought he was joking, until I asked one of his friends if it was true. Maybe he was embarrassed by the title, and maybe a little shy—like Clark Kent turning into Superman. (Would I love the true man or his disguise?) "Prince" is a loaded word too. He preferred just being Adriano. He preferred a girl like me, who worked her way through school, who knew the value of things and didn't put up with nonsense, didn't care who owned what or didn't. Like all of us, he wanted to be loved for himself.

And what about me? I was upset when I found out. Adriano was someone else than I had imagined. I felt confused. Prince of the Holy Roman Empire? What did that even mean?

"Relax," my mother said. "It's just a title. You're not going to turn into Princess Diana. You've got no kingdom to rule. Only one thing matters: do you love him?"

Of course I did, but at that point I was overwhelmed. Adriano had become someone new, mysterious, like dating a stranger. He hadn't really lied. Neither had he told the truth—until now. It was like Zorro taking off his mask.

"Let me get this straight," my sister Marisa said. "You're okay if he's from a Mafia family, but not if he's a prince?"

Our backgrounds were as opposite as they came. My family rarely had money. My parents were adventurers. They travelled the world performing, mostly on a thin dime. They busked in the Paris metros and also sang on French TV. Later, they owned a popular bar in southern Spain. I was born in Italy, my sister in Madrid, and my brother on Spain's Costa del Sol. Our fortunes were up and down, but my parents always found a way to make anywhere we lived home. Life was about attitude, not money. In that wisdom, I grew up wealthy beyond belief.

Adriano Pignatelli Aragona Cortes, Prince of the Holy Roman Empire, was heir to a thousand-year lineage that included kings of Sicily and Spain; Catherine of Aragon, wife of King Henry VIII; bishops and cardinals and even a pope—Innocent XII, along with a bona fide saint—Joseph Pignatelli. Though I was more impressed when he told me that his parents had vacationed with Jackie O, Princess Grace and Audrey Hepburn.

Adriano proposed on Christmas Eve a year later, and we were married in royal fashion on July 3, 1999, in London. A chauffeured Rolls Royce. The historic Farm Street Church in Mayfair filled with friends, family and the heady fragrance of Casablanca lilies.

My gown was raw silk, off the shoulder. The full skirt was delicately finished with a gorgeous sweeping train. One of my favorite things about it was its cost: $600. Though Adriano's generous mother had offered to buy me any gown I wanted at her expense, and even fly me to New York to go shopping, I wasn't willing to have her pay for something I couldn't buy for myself. I found my gown in a regular bridal store in Los Angeles. I liked its understated simplicity. It needed only a few finishing touches to make it perfect. I glue-gunned silk gardenias to the bustle, and made the bridal veil myself.

I swore I wouldn't cry. In fact, tears had been strongly discouraged by Susan, my new mother-in-law and head princess of the Pignatelli family, who possessed a certain sense of decorum, along with the very practical motive of what would look good in the photo shoot after-wards. Susan had designed the whole exquisite wedding, start to fin-ish, with the meticulous perfection of both commando general and haute couturier. I didn't want to let her down.

So of course, when the priest said, "Ivana, do you take Adriano Pignatelli Aragona Cortes to be your lawful wedded husband?" I shook,

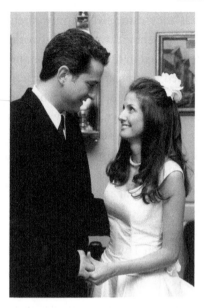

sobbing quietly at first, then sniffling, tearing, almost choking. Oh, the silence in the church as I tried to pull myself together! The priest awaited my reply.

Marisa—my sister, maid of honor, and best friend—leaned over and whispered: "Why did the chicken cross the road?" The unfunniest joke in the world, but her timing was perfect. We both got the giggles and I said, "I do."

We honeymooned in Capri, Monte Carlo, and Spain. What can I say? Sometimes fairytales do come true.

Adriano and I were married for ten years before we decided to have a baby. I was 34 years old. We had done everything we had planned to in our first years of marriage—a life mixed with exotic adventures and down-home goodness. We travelled the world. Yachting on the Mediterranean. Dining with ambassadors. Feasting in India with the Maharaja of Jodhpur one memorable New Year's Eve, complete with jeweled elephants, blazing fireworks and Bollywood-style dancers. We bought a home big enough for three. I had recently gotten my Masters in Education and was a successful consultant. Adriano's businesses were taking off. It seemed there was nothing we couldn't do if we just planned thoroughly enough and stuck to our Spreadsheet of Life.

I immediately became pregnant the first month of trying. A sweet surprise for us both. Between weeks seven and eight, I suffered a miscarriage. Adriano and I were devastated, but took some comfort as the doctor explained that miscarriage was nature's way of making sure only the healthiest babies made it to full term.

The doctor told us we had to wait until my body was back on its normal cycle, then add two-to-three months after the cycle normalized to begin trying again.

Six months later, my bio-clock was in high gear. Planning was everything, that's what I figured. Timing, yes. I bought an ovulation kit, measured my LH (luteinizing hormones), counted the days. We scheduled romance. *Every 14th day after the first day of my period.* Clockwork love. We did everything right and yet…

Five months passed. No baby. I went to a specialist recommended by a friend of mine for some testing.

On Christmas Eve day, the fertility specialist told me and my husband that we were candidates for in vitro. According to the tests, only a small percentage of my eggs were "good."

The rest? Failures, I supposed, as I listened to the doctor explain why women in their thirties had lower fertility rates, going down each decade from there; why my low Inhibin B hormone pretty much gave me a next-to-nil chance of getting pregnant the old-fashioned way, though he concluded his diagnosis by saying, "Ultimately, it's in the hands of something bigger than you or me."

What was the "something bigger?" I wondered. God or aging?

My father and sister were visiting for the holidays. I could barely stand to tell them the news. I had expected to give them a better gift. Papa said, "It's great. The good thing is that you will be able to have a baby. The results are the same." It was just like my father to put a positive spin on something that made my heart ache. We were in the kitchen. I turned away and started doing the dishes. It was just like me to bury what I felt, to stay busy and keep it all inside, but I couldn't. I started to cry.

"It is *not* great!" I shouted. "My body isn't doing what it's supposed to do. I've already lost one child and now my body isn't working again." All the fears of my bio-clock not just slowing down, but breaking completely, raged against my now elusive dream of motherhood.

Marisa hugged me. "I know you are going to have a baby, no matter what anyone says." She'd had a dream the night before: I was sitting at the dining room table drinking apple juice. In the dream, Marisa asked me why I wasn't having wine. I looked at her as though she were an idiot and said, "Because I'm pregnant." We looked up the meaning in a dream dictionary. Apple is a symbol of fertility.

Little did I know that very Christmas Eve, despite the doctor's bad news and my own inconsolable sorrow, I was already pregnant.

Chapter 2

Will I Ever Be the Same?

I was cautious the first few months of pregnancy, given my previous miscarriage. I went to acupuncture once a week for the first trimester and took homeopathic supplements to help with blood circulation to the uterus. My goal was to be as healthy as possible for me and the baby. That meant working out, eating right, getting plenty of sleep, and having a happy, relaxed attitude and disposition—despite nausea, fatigue and the emotional-hormonal rollercoaster ride of a lifetime.

So that was my plan. Reality: relax? What is that in this modern world? My days consisted of a full work load at the office, in addition to running a household; shopping, meal prep and the hundred other things you can't even put into a list, or remember when the day is done—especially now that you're pregnant. Maybe it is nature's wisdom—the hormonal amnesia that sets in, forcing you to let go of the non-essentials. My fondness for lists and organization took a new turn. Priorities shifted.

Pregnancy transforms you. Love your body through all its changes.

My body was writing new rules. I had little choice but to sit up and listen.

Redefining Beauty

Pregnancy forces you to redefine beauty in your own terms. Talk about growth! It is not just your baby who is growing. It is you, and I don't mean your belly or multiplying waist size. You, the core woman.

Weight gain, belly bump, plump rosy ankles—all the nagging body-image details a woman does her best to avoid become beautiful, even meaningful, in the bloom of new life. You are fertile, not fat. Learning to love your body through all its changes is a remarkable process.

And then there are the other changes, more of an animal nature. These include hair in strange places, bloating, farting, constipation, swelling and the desire to sing madly at the top of your lungs. The uterus can expand up to five hundred times its size. Feet can grow by a size or two. Okay, I love my body but really, Mother Nature, what gives?

When I first noticed the downy beard on my left cheek, I was on my way to an over-the-top party. Dressed to the nines, every hair in place—except for the new ones sprouting on only one side of my face. I was in a hurry and had no idea what to do. I decided to wax it. I prepped the wax strips, pressed hard and pulled with a firm yank. That ought to do it.

As I bent over to squeeze into my embellished gladiator sandals (the hot style for that season), I realized my ankles had turned into cankles! Where *had* my ankles gone? I grunted, stretching the strap to the last hole possible, only to notice another new development: an itchy red rash where my beard used to be.

In the car, I wore an icepack on my cheek. Adriano asked me why I didn't wax sooner, instead of right before the party. How could I explain that my beard had appeared almost magically overnight, that my body was doing whatever it pleased, whenever it pleased, and I seemed to be the last to know.

I smeared on thick makeup, but the rash still shined through. My last-ditch solution: I tossed my hair over the left side of my face and pretended it was on purpose—my sultry new look.

At the party, I mingled with the other guests, mocktail in hand. My feet felt heavy, swollen and clinking in black leather and gold hardware. I just hoped my sandals weren't going to burst any minute and blind someone with gold shrapnel.

All Things Will Pass

There is no one-size-fits-all pregnancy. Every woman is different, and how her body responds to pregnancy is as varied as human nature. Some lucky women breeze through the whole nine months with barely a symptom; while most of us will experience, in varying degrees, the common signals of new motherhood. Morning sickness, enhanced sense of smell, cravings, aversions and all the rest have real biological reasons beyond just making you sometimes feel like a stranger in your own body. Being stressed about these changes only makes them seem bigger. Pregnancy is a relatively short time, if you take the long view of life. Forty weeks. It helps to look at it in trimesters. Each trimester has its own unique aspects and symptoms.

A trimester is roughly three months. I figure I can handle anything for that length of time. By the time you master the ups and downs, you're on to a new stage. (This is also a good mindset for your baby's first year, to see you through the transitions of newborn development.)

The first trimester ushers in your transformation. You get to know yourself and your body in new ways. The baby makes its presence felt. Breasts are tender, a gnawing in the tummy, exhaustion, hunger, nausea, a sense something has shifted—drastically, which can feel similar to severe PMS. You will need several hours more sleep each night, but insomnia is also common due to hormonal changes. Euphoria, elations, humiliations, push-you-to-the-wall anger, amnesia and obstinance are all part of new motherhood, not to mention gas from both ends.

Yes, one of the most common pregnancy fears during the first trimester is wondering if you are going to *let one rip tater chip* in a meeting with co-workers. Just about the time you think you can't take any more of this, the second trimester begins.

The second trimester gives you back your energy, your sex drive, and some of the aspects of the old you. You've also been through the worst of the nausea.

Things are looking up. It's a good time to take those classes on pregnancy and birthing, set up your birth plan, and get your home ready for the new arrival.

In the third trimester, the baby's growing presence takes center stage. Your body may feel like it's being crowded out by the star of the show. (It is.) Your baby's most rapid weight gain will happen during this time. You'll feel her movements. She knows your voice, can open her eyes, and even see light. The reality of parenthood begins to set in as childbirth draws near. Emotions toggle between elation and anxiety.

No matter the challenges. You are so close to touchdown, there is a quiet joy in all that is taking place.

Knowing what's coming helps. Happily there is more information at our fingertips than ever before. The only problem, there's so much knowledge out there, it could become a full-time job just to find it! That's where I come in: I've done the work for you. What follows is an easy reference to the essentials for a happy, healthy pregnancy.

Chapter 3

Healthy Eats

The best advice on diet and nutrition is: relax. Encourage yourself to make the necessary changes for you and your baby's health. Start from where you are, wherever that is, and do your best.

During your first trimester, if you were at a healthy pre-pregnancy weight, your baby should be growing fine without too many dietary shifts. Recommended caloric increase is only 150-200 calories a day (about 1 cup of low fat yogurt). Don't sweat it on the scales. A gain of just a few pounds over the first few months is normal. Likewise if you gain more, don't worry. Eat well and stay active.

In the second and third trimesters, consistent weight gain is more important, and you have to eat more. Recommended caloric increase bumps up to 300 calories a day. Expect to gain about 3-4 pounds a month, if you began at a healthy pre-pregnancy weight. If underweight, you may need a larger caloric boost. If overweight, your doctor may recommend a slightly lower caloric increase. Counting calories is not as important as eating well and staying active. Don't stress about eating or gaining. Do your best, work with your doctor, and things will balance out.

> Eat an average of 300 more calories a day during your second and third trimesters.

My friend Jill had a history of eating disorders. She said the greatest lesson pregnancy taught her was to learn to listen to her body. Are you hungry? Eat. Stop dieting! In our overly image-conscious society, low birth-weight is a real issue.

Weight Gain: What is Right for You

Healthy babies are born to women of all shapes and sizes. Weight is not the only factor for a good pregnancy, but gaining too much or too little can result in health risks for both mother and baby. Recommended weight gain depends upon your weight prior to pregnancy, according to the National Academy of Sciences. In assessing your pre-pregnancy weight, take into account your BMI (body mass index), which is based upon weight and height.

You can calculate your BMI at www.nhlbisupport.com/bmi.

Weight Gain

Pre-pregnancy Weight	BMI	Recommended Weight Gain
Underweight	less than 18.5	28—40 pounds
Normal Weight	18.5 to 24.9	25—35 pounds
Overweight	25 to 29.9	15—25 pounds
Obese	30 or greater	11—20 pounds

Institute of Medicine

Where does the new weight go? The baby contributes 7-8 pounds. Another 7 pounds goes to maternal fat stores (fat stores help fuel the baby's development; unused fat stores switch to boosting mom's energy during lactation). Breasts grow by 2 pounds, as does the uterus. Maternal blood volume is increased by 3-4 pounds. Increased fluid volume, another 3-4 pounds. Placenta, 1-2 pounds. Amniotic fluid, 2 pounds.

Nutrition Essentials

Do your best to make healthy choices. Avoid alcohol. Eat plenty of fresh vegetables and fruit, lean protein, and whole grains. Good nutrition applies now more than ever. Your baby is eating whatever you eat. If you are eating healthy, your baby has a better chance of being healthy too. By the 5th week of pregnancy, your baby's heart, brain, organs and spinal cord begin to form. Nutrient-rich foods are your baby's building blocks, and will affect your child throughout her/his life. It makes sense to make peace with any necessary changes.

If you find yourself struggling, think of it this way: nutritious foods give more of the good fat your body needs for energy and less of the bad fat that lands on your hips and clogs your arteries. Not only that, you get better looking. Good nutrition makes your hair shine, gives your skin radiance, and boosts your emotional well-being. What's not to like?

On the other side, junk food increases the risk of gestational diabetes and other complications that are best avoided.

Five Nutrients You Can't Do Without

Pay special attention to these top five nutrients essential for a healthy pregnancy.

Key Nutrients	
Folate and folic acid (800 mcg a day)	Prevents birth defects. Spinach, beans, asparagus, peas, peanuts, oranges, & cereal
Calcium (1000 mg a day)	Strengthens bones; fuels circulatory, muscular and nervous systems. Milk, cheese, cottage cheese, yogurt, salmon, spinach, cereal, calcium-fortified orange juice
Vitamin D (600 IU a day)	Builds baby's bones & teeth. Asparagus, eggs, milk, salmon, tuna, vitamin D-fortified juice
Protein (71 grams a day) Especially essential 2nd and 3rd trimesters.	Promotes growth, builds cells and brain. Lean meat, poultry, fish, eggs, dried beans, peas, tofu, dairy products, peanut butter
Iron (27 mgs a day)	Prevents anemia, fatigue, promotes healthy blood supply to baby. The need for iron doubles in pregnancy. Lean red meat, poultry, fish, beans, spinach, iron-fortified cereal, nuts, dried fruit. For better absorption, combine with foods high in vitamin C.

Mayoclinic.com/pregnancy diet -USDA Nutrient Database for Standard Reference, Release 23

Simple Switches for Great Health

So you're not such a healthy eater. Who is? Now is the time to start. Begin with simple things: when you crave sugar, eat fruit. When you crave carbohydrates, eat whole grains instead of refined grains, which are less nutritious. Choose brown rice over white rice, whole oats over instant oatmeal. Whole fresh foods are always more nutritious than processed foods and will fill you up longer. Check your shopping list and substitute healthier choices for your kitchen staples:

Nutritious Choices	
BUY	**TO REPLACE**
Whole grain bread, pastas, cereals, rice	White bread, pastas, cereals, rice
Fresh fruits and vegetables	Canned fruits and vegetables
Think rainbow: the brighter the colors, the higher the nutrients. Mix colors: dark green leaf with orange and red veggies.	
Honey (pasteurized), real maple syrup	Corn syrup, artificial maple syrup
Healthy oils (high in monounsaturates/no trans fats)	Hydrogenated, high fat oils
Best oils: olive, sesame, walnut, avocado Worst oils: palm, cottonseed	
Skim milk 1%, no added hormones/antibiotics	Whole milk (high in fat)
If you are lactose intolerant or vegan, make sure your rice, almond, coconut or soy milks contain added calcium.	
Meats, poultry (no hormones, antibiotics, or nitrates)	Meats/poultry with added chemicals
Real fruit sodas, sparkling water	Sugary sodas or high-caffeine drinks
100% fruit and vegetable juices	Sugary juice cocktails
Iodized salt	Non-iodized salt
Only 70% of table salt is iodized. Check the label.	

The Importance of Iodine

Pregnant women need 50% more iodine than other adults. Iodine plays a crucial role in fetal brain and nervous system development. Low iodine can result in lower IQs in babies. The recommended dose for pregnant women is 220 mcg daily. Lactating moms need 290 mcg a day.

A good source of iodine is iodized table salt. You don't need much.

To get your 220 mcg of iodine requires roughly ½ heaping teaspoon of iodized salt a day. For lactating women, 290 mcg of iodine is equivalent to about ¾ teaspoon of iodized salt.

Buying Tips

- Many stores offer a bulk section where you can buy fresh nuts, whole grains, cereals, and flour at better prices than the pre-packaged items.

- Choose glass containers over cans and plastics. Most cans and plastics contain BPA, a hormone-disrupter linked to problems in fetal development.

- Just because an item is marketed as "natural" or "healthy" doesn't mean it's good for you. Check labels. Keep your eye out for unhealthy additives like MSG, high sugar or sodium, artificial coloring or flavors, nitrates, hydrogenated oils, trans fats, saturated fats.

The Skinny on Fat

There is good fat and bad fat. Bad fat: saturated and trans fats, which raise bad cholesterol and can lower good cholesterol. (An exception is the saturated fat (stearic acid) in dark chocolate that does not affect cholesterol.) Good fat: unsaturated fats, which are essential fatty acids your body needs for energy.

"Most of the fat that you eat should come from unsaturated sources: polyunsaturated fats and monounsaturated fats. In general, nuts, vegetable oils, and fish are sources of unsaturated fats" (Centers for Disease Control and Prevention). Check out the table below for specific examples of unsaturated fats.

Healthy Fats		
Monounsaturated Fat Sources	Omega-6 Polyunsaturated Fat Sources	Omega-3 Polyunsaturated Fat Sources
Nuts Vegetable oils Canola oil Olive oil High oleic safflower oil Sunflower oil Avocado	Soybean oil Corn oil Safflower oil	Soybean oil Canola oil Walnuts Flaxseed Fish: trout, herring, and salmon

Centers for Disease Control and Prevention (CDC)

Craving Fixes

Many doctors believe pregnancy cravings are simply your body's way of telling you what you need, unless you are craving cream-filled donuts with double-fudge icing 24 hours a day. A lot of women crave sugar because the body needs extra energy. But pregnancy is not an invitation to eat as much junk as you want, since you're going to gain anyway. Though I've got to say, *having* to eat more food *is* fun.

Do what works and don't feel guilty. If you want a piece of chocolate cake, eat it. Indulge with pleasure when you do. Balance cravings with common sense. (Have one, not five.) Dark chocolate is good for you in moderate amounts, thanks to its high antioxidants and lower sugar content. Savor the flavor. Keep portions small.

Listen to your strong aversions too. If something turns you off, don't eat it, even if it's healthy or was your favorite munchy ever since you were a kid. Tastebuds change, especially in the first trimester. You may dislike foods you used to love or experience an increased sensitivity to bitter tastes, among other foodie surprises. Common pregnancy cravings for sour, salty, spicy and sweet help balance out the bitter factor. Why do tastebuds go rogue? Fluctuating estrogen levels play a part and will even out by second trimester.

If you feel you aren't getting the nutrients you need due to nausea or aversions, be sure you are taking your prenatals, which should ideally start 3 months before you conceive, and all the way through breastfeeding. (For more on prenatal vitamins, see page 27.)

Sugar Facts

Our bodies need glucose (blood sugar) to fuel our cells, brain and other organs. Carbohydrates in fruits, vegetables and whole grains are the best sources of glucose. It can also come from sugar. But we don't need much. How much? Six teaspoons a day for women, according to the American Heart Association. The average American eats 22 teaspoons a day!

Which is better—honey or sugar? Dark molasses, honey, maple syrup and raw sugar have higher antioxidants and are healthier alternatives to refined sugar, corn syrup and agave nectar (*Journal of the American Dietetic Association*). The difference is the equivalent of a serving of nuts or berries a day. But even with healthier alternatives, low sugar recommendations still apply.

Nutritionally and calorie-wise there is little difference between brown sugar and white sugar. Most brown sugar is white refined sugar with molasses added.

Artificial Sweeteners. Products labeled "sugar-free" often have artificial sweeteners. According to the FDA, most are considered safe in moderation during pregnancy. But Dr. Andrew Weil advises everyone, pregnant or not: "Skip the artificial sweeteners. They are unhealthy and don't help you develop good eating habits." If you are diabetic, talk to your doctor about healthy sugar substitutes.

Quick & Easy: Ways to Cut Sugar

1 One-half teaspoon of cinnamon a day can lower blood sugar by 25%.

2 In baking recipes, cut sugar in half and sweeten with cinnamon, natural vanilla, or nutmeg.

3 Stop drinking sugar sodas, which have 10 teaspoons of sugar in a single can. Try low-sugar natural sodas instead.

Fish and Pregnancy: You Need It!

Fish is a crucial part of a healthy pregnancy diet. The omega-3 fatty acids found in seafood promote healthy brain development in your baby. Fish is also a good source of protein and iron—critical building blocks for your baby's growth and developing nervous system.

How much fish should I eat? The FDA and EPA recommend that a pregnant woman consume 12 ounces of fish per week, which is equivalent to two meals. Other studies show an increased benefit from eating seafood at least three times a week.

Wild or farm-raised? Wild-caught is preferable to farm-raised. If eating local fish, pay attention to local fish advisories.

What about mercury? Not all fish are created equal. Large predatory fish contain higher levels of mercury, so avoid shark, swordfish, king mackerel and tilefish. Other types of fish contain little or no mercury. Plan your meals from this list of low-mercury seafood: salmon, pollock, tilapia, catfish, shrimp, cod, crab, canned light tuna (NOT albacore or ahi; both have high mercury levels).

But I hate seafood! If you are allergic to seafood, vegan or just can't stand the taste, be sure to get your omega-3 fatty acids in some other form. Flax and fish oil are good sources. Choose a fish oil that contains EPA (eicosapentaenoic acid) and DHA (docosahexaenoic acid), two of the most important omega-3s for optimum health.

Foods to Avoid

Pregnant women are at higher risk for foodborne bacterial illnesses. With *E. coli* on the rise, it's good practice for anyone to wash all fruits and vegetables thoroughly. It takes heat to kill bacteria and parasites that could harm the baby. That's why the FDA and EPA recommend pregnant and nursing women avoid:

- Unpasteurized milk, juices, and soft cheeses
    - Soft cheeses include feta, blue cheese, brie, camembert, queso blanco, queso fresco and panela. Pasteurized versions of these cheeses exist. Check the label. If marked "pasteurized," it is fine to eat.

- Undercooked or raw meat, seafood, shellfish, eggs. (No sushi or carpaccio.)

  - Undercooked meat includes deli meats such as bologna, hot dogs, ham, turkey and salami. Cook until steaming hot throughout.
  - Undercooked seafood includes refrigerated smoked fish, such as lox. Cook until steaming hot throughout.
  - Pre-stuffed poultry makes the list, along with refrigerated pates and meat spreads. Heat thoroughly. Cook poultry stuffing separately to 165°. Frozen pre-stuffed poultry is safe, when cooked from frozen state. Cook eggs until firm throughout. Avoid eggnog or any raw egg product.
  - Raw cookie dough or cake batter
  - Raw sprouts

Buying Guide

When Should I Buy Organic?

What is "organic" anyway? Simply put, organic produce is non-GMO, grown without pesticides, chemical fertilizers, sewage sludge (yes, sewage), bioengineering or radiation. Organic poultry, meat, eggs and dairy products come from animals that aren't given antibiotics or growth hormones. Organic farmers keep the soil nutrient-rich through sustainable farming. Good for our kids, good for the planet. The growing consensus among scientists is that pesticides on produce can affect human health, especially during fetal development and early childhood.

Go organic for meat, dairy, coffee, poultry, eggs and baby foods.

It makes sense to buy organic. But if you are on a budget—and who isn't these days?—organics can be expensive. You don't always have to buy organic. Some conventional products are fine, as long as they contain low-pesticide residue.

Consumer Reports recommends going organic for meat, dairy, coffee, poultry, eggs and baby foods. For produce, check out the Environmental Working Group's *Dirty Dozen and Clean Fifteen*. EWG sets the gold standard each year with their shoppers' guide of the highest pesticide produce and lowest pesticide produce, compiled from analysis of over 89,000 tests.

Dirty Dozen/Clean Fifteen

Dirty Dozen High pesticides Buy organic	Clean Fifteen Low pesticides Conventional ok
1. Apples (worst)	1. Onions (best)
2. Celery	2. Sweet corn
3. Sweet bell peppers	3. Pineapples
4. Peaches	4. Avocado
5. Strawberries	5. Cabbage
6. Nectarines (imported)	6. Sweet peas
7. Grapes	7. Asparagus
8. Spinach	8. Mangoes
9. Lettuce	9. Eggplant
10. Cucumbers	10. Kiwi
11. Blueberries (domestic)	11. Cantaloupe (domestic)
12. Potatoes	12. Sweet potatoes
Plus: Green beans &	13. Grapefruit
Kale/greens	14. Watermelon
	15. Mushrooms

Farmers' Markets and CSAs

Buy local and buy seasonal if you want to get fresh, healthy food at the best prices. Farmers' markets are a good source. With over 7,000 operating in the U.S., there is a good chance you may find one near you. Fun for the whole family, many farmers' markets are a combination of arts, live music and fresh food, with plenty of free samples. A great place to try out new tastes. You'll find me at my local farmers market every Sunday morning, where I can eat breakfast, do the shopping and let my kids play—all at the same time.

Just because it's a farmers' market, doesn't mean it's all organic. Organic produce will be clearly marked. If it doesn't say organic, it's probably not.

Another good option in many communities is to join a CSA (Community Supported Agriculture). Customers buy a set price share or subscription direct from the farmer. In return, each week you receive a fresh box of the season's harvest. The fresher the food, the richer nutrients.

Breakfast

A Great Day

We've all heard it before: breakfast is the most important meal of the day. A good breakfast will fuel you through the morning, improve focus and creativity, and lower cholesterol and stress. Not only that, adults who eat breakfast tend to eat more vitamins and less fat. Probably because when we miss breakfast, hunger strikes mid-morning, and we rush out to the nearest burrito wagon or pastry shop and devour everything in sight!

Super Starts
- Hot oatmeal with raisins, almonds or dried cranberries.

- Whole grain cereal with skim milk or low-fat yogurt.

- Fruit smoothie with low-fat yogurt. Try super antioxidant mango and blueberries.

- Peanut butter on whole grain toast or bagel.

- Eggs and veggie scramble. Try nutrient-rich broccoli, avocado or red peppers.

Mini-Meals

Pregnant women need to eat more often (4-6 times a day) and in smaller portions. This maintains energy levels and staves off nausea. If you are on the go a lot, it helps to pack a few snacks in your car, purse, and work place.

High Energy, Take Anywhere Snacks
- Go nuts. Best for health: almonds, walnuts, peanuts, pistachios.

- Dried fruits. A good alternative to candy. ½ cup dried fruit is equal to 1 cup fresh fruit.

- Cereal bars. Look for whole grain, low-fat, low-sugar.

My Anytime Favorites
- Peanut butter with apple slices

- Cheese and whole grain crackers

- Hummus and organic blue corn tortilla chips

- Low-fat yogurt and fresh fruit

Tummy Easers

If you are prone to nausea, ginger works wonders. Keep ginger snaps, ginger candy, low-sugar ginger ale or ginger tea on hand. To prevent morning sickness, try a combination of carbohydrates and proteins, like cheese and crackers. Yogurt is also a good tummy soother.

Gourmet Mama

Good nutrition should taste good too. Figure it this way: you are going to have to eat healthy, first for nine months and then six or so, if breastfeeding. A total of fifteen months. You might as well enjoy it and make it easy on yourself!

Lunch can be as simple as a quick spinach salad with pine nuts and cranberries; or a whole-grain tuna salad sandwich with avocadoes, tomatoes and a sprinkle of arugula leaves. Once a week, I buy a whole roast chicken. We have it for dinner with brown rice and steamed veggies, and use the chicken leftovers for lunch the next day, either in a red-lettuce salad or chicken pita pockets with hummus.

For dinner, I like a bit of elegance from time-to-time. Here are three of my favorite recipes for delicious, nutritious meals. Enjoy!

Simple Recipes

Dijon Salmon & Brown Rice

Ingredients (Serves 2)

- ☐ Salmon—1 lb. filet
- ☐ 1 jar of capers (4.4 oz/125 gram size)
- ☐ 4 to 5 medium tomatoes
- ☐ 8 spring onions
- ☐ 2 tablespoons white wine
- ☐ 1 tablespoon of Dijon mustard
- ☐ 2 cups brown rice

Salmon

1. Cook brown rice ahead of time. Follow directions on rice package as cooking times vary.

2. Preheat oven to 425°F.

3. Dice tomatoes and chop spring onions.

4. Spread mustard on top of the salmon. Layer spring onions on top. Then add a layer of diced tomatoes, followed by the capers. Splash with white wine. Salt and pepper to taste.

5. Bake for 20-25 minutes, depending on thickness of salmon filet.

6. Serve with steamed broccoli and brown rice. (Or steamed vegetables of your choice.)

Lemon Rosemary Chicken with Asparagus & Potatoes

Ingredients (serves 4)

- ☐ 4 skinless chicken breasts
- ☐ 2 tablespoons of olive oil
- ☐ 2 sprigs of rosemary (remove leaves, discard stems)
- ☐ 1 lemon
- ☐ Salt and pepper
- ☐ Asparagus bunch
- ☐ 8 small red potatoes

Cooking Directions: Chicken

1. Place the chicken breasts in a large Ziploc.
2. With a cooking hammer pound the chicken out thinly.
3. Add olive oil, juice from 1 lemon, rosemary sprigs, salt and pepper to the Ziploc bag.
4. Mix the marinade so it covers the chicken. Place in fridge and let it marinate for an hour.
5. Cook the chicken on the grill or frying pan with olive oil (about 4 minutes on each side or until the center is no longer pink).

Potatoes

1. Preheat the oven to 400°F.
2. Cut red potatoes into quarters and place on baking sheet.
3. Cover with olive oil. Sprinkle with salt & pepper.
4. Bake at 400 for 15-20 minutes. Stir frequently.

Asparagus

1. Wash the asparagus and cut off bottom quarter of stalk.
2. Sauté in olive oil in a fry pan (alternate: steam over water).
3. Season with salt & pepper and cover.
4. Cook for about 5 minutes, or until stalks pierce with a fork easily.

Tomato Leek Pasta
Tastes even better the next day!

Ingredients (serves 4)

- ☐ 8 medium ripe tomatoes
- ☐ 3 leeks
- ☐ 7 cloves of garlic
- ☐ ½ cup olive oil
- ☐ Salt
- ☐ Mozzarella (Note: mozzarella is a semi-soft pasteurized cheese, which is fine for pregnancy. Do not use buffalo mozzarella, which sometimes is not pasteurized. Check the label.)
- ☐ 1 box of Barilla thick spaghetti

Cooking Directions

1. Put olive oil in a saucepan, along with 7 cloves of garlic and a pinch of salt. Simmer over a low to medium heat.

2. Brown the garlic and remove it from the pan.

3. Cut leeks into thin round slices and add them to the oil. Cook leeks for 3 minutes.

4. Dice tomatoes into large chunks and add to leeks and olive oil. Add salt to taste.

5. Cook over a low flame for 2 to 3 hours, stirring occasionally.

6. Follow the Barilla spaghetti cooking instruction. Once water boils, pasta takes about 10 minutes to cook.

7. Mix sauce with spaghetti. Sprinkle mozzarella on top and enjoy!

Chapter 4

Daily Essentials

Prenatal Vitamins

Most doctors recommend prenatal vitamins in addition to a nutrient-rich diet. You don't have to go the expensive prescription route. There are many good over-the-counter brands. You may have to try out a few before you find the one that works for you. Most doctors can provide samples. You will have to take them throughout your pregnancy and on into postpartum (especially if you choose to breastfeed), so find a good fit.

Prenatal vitamins generally contain higher amounts of folic acid, calcium, and iron than regular vitamins—all vital to the baby's development.

According to the Mayo Clinic, here's what to look for in a prenatal vitamin:

Folic acid—400-800 micrograms	Zinc—15 milligrams
Calcium—250 milligrams	Copper—2 milligrams
Iron—30 milligrams	Vitamin B6—2 milligrams
Vitamin C—30 milligrams	Vitamin D—400 IU

Diet also plays a part in what your body needs. If you are not drinking enough milk, you may need additional calcium. If you are anemic, you will need more iron. If you are not eating enough fish, you may need more omega-3s or iodine.

Only half of prenatal vitamins sold in the U.S. contain iodine. You may need iodine supplements if you are not getting the recommended dose (220 mcg daily) through iodine-rich foods; lactating moms need 290 mcg daily. Talk with your healthcare provider about your best choices.

Balance is the key. Take all supplements as prescribed. Though vitamin A is important, high doses can cause birth defects. What is the right amount of vitamin A? About 770 micrograms daily during pregnancy. If you are eating enough fruits and vegetables, you should be getting plenty of vitamin A without taking a supplement.

- If you forget to take your vitamins, don't double up. Take the normal amount the following day.

- If you have morning sickness, try taking your prenatal vitamins at night, with food.

Water

Your body is made up mostly of water. During pregnancy, it is all the more important to stay hydrated with 10 glasses of fluids a day (78 oz.). Breastfeeding women need 13 glasses of fluids a day (105 oz.). Though coffee, teas, juice and soft drinks count toward that goal, some of these are high in sugar or caffeine which require limited intake during pregnancy. Water is by far the best hydration for your body.

If you're not used to drinking a lot of water, try sprucing it up with a slice of lime or lemon, or a splash of fresh juice. Make your own soda by adding juice to sparkling water. Refresh: add fresh mint, cucumber or strawberries to a pitcher of cool water.

Try to work water into your daily routines. Buy a stainless steel bottle and stay hydrated wherever you go. It's more effective to drink smaller amounts of water more often, than waiting until you're thirsty, then guzzling to meet your quota. Hydration works best, same as your snacks, sprinkled throughout the day.

Some women fear that drinking a lot of water will contribute to water retention and cankles. This is a myth. Staying hydrated actually helps prevent water retention. Hydration signals your body that you are getting enough water, and therefore do not need to hold onto it.

Safe Drinking Water

What does "safe" drinking water mean? More than 80% of tap water in U.S. cities contains varying levels of contaminants, but is still safe to drink if you have no health problems. Pregnant women and children are more vulnerable to health risks imposed by even low levels of contaminants. Water filters are a simple solution.

A recent tap-water study of 35 U.S. cities, showed 31 had unsafe chromium-6 levels.Chromium-6 is the toxin made famous in the movie *Erin Brockovich*, known to cause cancer and other ailments. If you happen to live in one of these cities (as I do—in Los Angeles), drink only filtered water and use it for cooking, as well as in your baby's formula. (Boiling only increases toxin concentrations.) The most effective filtration system for chromium-6 is reverse osmosis. It can be installed under your sink, and will last a decade if maintained properly.

Bottled water is not a solution, as it is often just repackaged tap water. There are many types of water filters available starting at $30. Your best choice of filter depends on what is in your water and what you are trying to filter out. For more information on safe water and filter options, including what's in your local water, check out Environmental Working Group at www.ewg.org.

To Tea or Not to Tea?

Herbal teas are generally not recommended during pregnancy. Why? There is not enough data on how herbs affect the developing fetus. A few teas are considered safe in moderate amounts: ginger tea is recommended by many health practitioners to alleviate nausea and boost the immune system. Other safe teas are peppermint, lime blossom, rose hips, and roasted barley.

Green and black teas are fine in moderate amounts. Just watch the caffeine. Healthy caffeine intake during pregnancy is less than 200 mg. a day, which is the equivalent of 2 cups of 8 oz. coffee or 4 cups of 8 oz. black or green tea.

The rest are best avoided, including teas marketed for pregnancy, and common teas such as chamomile, anise, hibiscus, lemongrass, licorice root, raspberry leaf, and sassafras.

Exercise

Working out may be one of the last things you want to think about when you are bloated, nauseous or fatigued. But for healthy pregnant women, 30 minutes a day of moderate exercise is recommended. Regular exercise will give you energy, keep you in shape and prepare you for labor. It helps with aches, pains, constipation, and fatigue. Another plus: exercise releases endorphins, the body's feel-good chemical. Great for managing hormonal mood swings. A half-hour walk a day will help you sleep better too.

Drink 1-2 cups of water for every half-hour of moderate exercise.

Be sure to check with your healthcare provider about any exercise routine you start, especially if you have had a prior miscarriage or other medical conditions. Always listen to your body.

If you worked out regularly before pregnancy, you should be able to continue at the same level of activity. Doctors used to think that keeping the heart rate below 140 beats a minute was important, but that thinking has changed. For healthy pregnant women, the U.S. Department of Health and Human Services now recommends "at least 2 hours and 30 minutes of moderate-intensity aerobic activity a week," spread throughout the week, without specific heart rate limits.

If you're not used to working out, start slow. Begin with five minutes a day, then ten, until you've worked your way up to thirty. Know when you are pushing too hard. If you can't speak normally, that's your body talking, telling you to slow down. Pace yourself. Stay hydrated. Drink an extra 1-2 cups of water for every half-hour of moderate exercise. If your body says *take it easy*, take it easier. Stay in touch with your doctor throughout pregnancy about any changes in your activity levels.

Build exercise into your daily routine. Choose a time that works best—meaning a time you are less likely to flake out. For me, it was a morning walk around the block. Easy. No planning. Just step outside the door. I didn't even have to be awake! That way, I got my exercise in before I went to work. I knew if I gave myself small goals, I would be more likely to take the first step. If I didn't get my walk in first thing, no matter how good my intentions, I never got around to it later in the day.

If you need extra motivation, find a partner or sign up for a class. Swimming, dance and stationary bicycles are also recommended forms of exercise for most pregnant women.

Many fitness centers offer prenatal exercise classes, including yoga. Hatha (gentle) yoga is best for new mothers. Avoid Bikram yoga, and any exercises that make you lie on your back.

Also avoid hot tubs and saunas. Core body temperature should not exceed 102°F (10 minutes in a hot tub). High temperatures can affect your blood pressure, and in turn your baby's oxygen supply.

For soothing renewal, go for a walk in nature. Cedars and pines release phytoncides, which strengthen the immune system and lower stress hormones. Natural surroundings also expose you to the soil microbe, *Mycobacterium vaccae*, which acts as both a calming agent and anti-depressant. You don't have to trek into the High Sierras to get your green workout. Brief walks in nature or parks are still beneficial, especially if water is nearby.

My all-time favorite exercise is dancing. An all-over feel-good experience you can do alone, with friends, even with your kids. As a friend of mine said, "There's no way to feel sad when you're dancing." Uplifting dance music increases your antibodies and lowers stress. Make a playlist of your favorites to have on hand whenever you need a boost.

Last but not least: don't forget your Kegel's. Tightening and releasing your pelvic floor muscles will help incontinence and bladder issues during pregnancy, and believe it or not, can also improve orgasm. These can be done anywhere, anytime. Contract and hold your pelvic floor for 5 seconds, then relax for 5 seconds. The goal is to reach an optimal 10 second contract/10 second relax cycle. Work your way up to 3 sets of 10 per day.

The Happiness Factor

Fun, pleasure, and play are a big part of health. A happy person lives approximately nine years longer than an unhappy person. It's better for you to eat a piece of your favorite chocolate cake loving every bite, than to rigidly sacrifice by eating only "what is good for you." One of my pregnancy cravings was a triple-layer coconut cake, which I ate the night before my son, Alessio, was born. It is also one of his favorite desserts. Strange but true: not only do babies in womb pick up on their mother's emotions, they also develop a preference for whatever mama was eating during pregnancy. All the more reason to eat well, enjoy life and your momentous transformation.

Quick & Easy: Ways to Stay Healthy

1   Drink 10 glasses of water a day.
    (Preferably filtered water vs. bottled.)

2   Get 30 minutes of moderate exercise a day.

3   Take your prenatal vitamins.

4   Eat smaller, more frequent meals (4-6 per day).
    Eat whole grains, organic produce and plenty of fish.

5   Keep a low-fat cereal bar in your bag
    when you're on the go.

6   Get at least 8 hours sleep a night.

7   Listen to your body. If you're tired, sleep.
    If you're hungry, eat.

Ten-minute Stress Cures

- Dance! Anywhere, anytime. Put on your favorite music and let loose.

- Laugh! Laughter is contagious and good for you. It relaxes muscles, boosts energy and strengthens your immune system. Go ahead, watch comedies. Give yourself a big laugh—even if you're alone, even if you're faking it to start—it works.

- Breathe! Let's face it: breathing can be boring. Maybe that's why it's so relaxing. Close your eyes and imagine an ocean or lake—or whatever gives you a feeling of calm. Stay with it while you breathe in *peace*, breathe out *stress*. Hold it there, a minute or two beyond your rush to get back to work. Understand that taking time for yourself is never a *waste* of time, but rather a *wealth* of time.

Things to Toss: Shame, fear, anxiety, guilt, self-censorship, perfectionism.

Things to Multiply: Laughter, self-esteem, relaxation, pleasure, health, love.

Chapter 5

Look Good, Feel Great!

First Rule of Beauty: Be Yourself. Or as Dolly Parton famously said, "Find out who you are, then do it on purpose."

My friend, Gabby, was pregnant with her first baby when her husband's grandmother invited her to go shopping at a "fat ladies store."

"I'm pregnant, Grandma, not fat," she said.

"No, you are fat," Granny insisted.

Later that night, Gabby told her husband, "I don't care if your grandmother *is* ninety, you'd better put her in check."

Gabby's husband never once told her that she was beautiful during her pregnancy. He's now her ex, and no wonder! Women have to be told they're beautiful when they are pregnant. Not only because they are beautiful, but fragile too. At times you begin to forget what you look like—strangely lost inside your ever-changing body. Every woman needs loving emotional support throughout pregnancy. This can come from friends, family and close social networks.

Ideally it should also come from your partner. If you are not getting the support you need, it's time to sit down and have a conversation. Tell him how you feel and what you would like from him. Be willing to listen too. To be fair, a lot of guys are nervous about pregnancy and don't know what to do, especially as they watch their wives' hormonal rollercoaster ride.

Some men are turned off (even scared) by the changes in their partner's body, while others are aroused and exhilarated. To turn that around, women often don't feel that sexy—especially as the baby grows bigger. And some women have an increased sex drive. Heightened sensitivity comes from increased blood flow to the hoo ha, love bits, or whatever name you prefer to call your privates. In this case, the ladies often outpace their men in the bedroom, which can create its own partnership insecurities. However you feel, be honest, loving and accepting of yourself.

When Gabby was pregnant with her second child (with her second husband), she was cleaning out her closet and came across the uniform she'd worn religiously during her first pregnancy: oversized T-shirts (gifts from her former in-laws). She held up the 3XXX-sized shirts, embroidered with Disney characters, and thought, "No wonder my ex never told me I was beautiful. Goofy, Mickey and Donald Duck aren't exactly Victoria's Secret."

Gabby decided then and there to make a conscious effort to feel beautiful and be beautiful. She bought sexy new clothes, had fun with her new curves, gave herself what she needed, when she needed it— whatever made her feel happy and good. It helped that she was with a man who recognized her true beauty—inside and out—and told her so.

Fashion Essentials

Fashion is fleeting but style is forever. Every woman knows what she feels comfortable in, and I don't mean sweatpants—though I've got my favorite pair. By comfortable, I mean style that is you. A big part of looking good is feeling confident in what you are wearing, and not having the clothes wear you. Though pregnancy can be a time of self-conscious body shifts, it is also the time when a woman comes into her own. Have fun with your new voluptuous figure. Show off your beautiful bump! Your wardrobe will need a few simple changes.

Start with comfortable fabric. Soft, breathable cottons or modals are best. Modal is softer, thinner and warmer than cotton and doesn't shrink. Layer up. Hot cold flashes–out of control! Be ready for ups and downs in body heat.

Colors that look good, make you feel great. We all have those colors that make our eyes pop, our skin glow. Wear anything that makes you smile.

Check out magazine covers when you are in the grocery line. Pay attention to the nail color being used, the way makeup has been applied, and the colors of the season. Window shop at your favorite boutique. Stores use mannequins to showcase the hottest styles. Most importantly: make any trend your own.

New Body Basics

You don't have to spend a lot of money on items you'll be growing into and out of, but there are certain things you'll be using so much, they are worth investing in.

Maternity Jeans: You will wear them at least four times a week, from second trimester to after delivery. It's worth spending a little more to get jeans that have the right style, fit and stretch. My favorites: JBrand and 7 for All Mankind.

Comfortable Shoes: Go for classic style and comfort. Find a pair with good arch support and supple leather that stretches if your feet expand. Pumps or ballet flats are easy to pair with any trend of clothing. Try a nude tone to elongate your legs, or basic black.

Long Dresses: Can't live without them! So comfortable and will keep you cool in hot weather. The floor-length hemline covered up my swollen ankles too. Keep the lines clean and sleek. Avoid puffy sleeves, or any style that makes you feel fluffier than you already do.

Fundamental Foundations

Camisoles with Built-in Shelf Bra: My favorite cami is Cosabella. I wear them day and night. They are perfect as a layering piece under tops that are a little too short, as well as being a super comfortable top to keep the girls in place. Pricey but worth it. If it is something you love and use a lot, don't be frugal with yourself. Be as comfortable as possible whenever possible.

Bellaband: Recommended for the first four months of pregnancy, the band allows you to wear your pants unbuttoned if they are non-maternity bottoms, and helps hide your bellybutton when it is stretched to the limits. Also stretches your wardrobe and budget by making up for tops that are a little too short!

Low-Rise Panties: Low-rise fit under your baby bump, rather than around it, maximizing comfort and minimizing adjustments.

New Bra: Your breasts are growing. Your husband is glowing. Of course you need a new bra! Maybe several over the 3 trimesters. Wireless bras are best for breast health. There are plenty of designs that offer great support. Any department store will fit you for your correct size.

Quick & Easy: Guilt-free Splurges

1   Pashmina or colorful scarves are my #1 must-have. Adds versatility, color and warmth to your wardrobe. Can be worn day or evening, whether you are dressed up or down. Also perfect for body temperature changes.

2   Fun scarves, bangles and bracelets, a cool pair of earrings. These are simple pleasures that don't depend on dress size, but can make any outfit work. Spice up your basics with a colorful pashmina or costume jewelry. Try something bold: a statement ring, a pop of color or something you have always wanted to try but never dared. Don't feel guilty about indulging yourself. Accessories can be worn after the baby is born.

3   Handbags always add an element of elegance. If you go large with lots of compartments, it can double as a diaper bag once the baby arrives.

4   Get an easy style update with a new pair of sunglasses. Go with a friend who is honest—the ultimate must-have.

Skin Deep

Radiant glow? Yes! For most moms-to-be, increased circulation creates a beautiful dewy freshness to the skin. But we can also experience acne, dry skin, dark patches, belly rash, skin tags, itching skin resulting from our once-firm bellies stretching to watermelon size. These are caused by hormonal changes and most will subside once your pregnancy ends. Be sure to use a good moisturizer and drink lots of water to stay hydrated. For dark patches, wear sunscreen to lessen pigmentation; use a good foundation or tinted moisturizer, and concealer where needed.

If you have acne (possibly even on your butt!), you can be thankful it's not as bad as those awkward teen years. Use a mild cleanser like oatmeal. Do not use Retin A or prescription acne treatments during pregnancy.

Spider veins, varicose veins and stretch marks are other skin changes most women experience to some degree. **Spider veins** are related to increased circulation and usually disappear after pregnancy.

Varicose veins are caused by increased pressure on the uterus, which increases pressure on the legs. For many women, varicose veins cause little or no discomfort. Others experience heaviness in the legs which can sometimes be painful. After delivery, things will ease up. In the meantime, you can lessen or prevent symptoms by walking, avoiding excessive weight gain, taking vitamin C, propping your feet up, sleeping on your left side for better circulation, and wearing maternity support hose. Varicose veins do shrink and can even disappear, about 3-4 months after delivery, especially if you didn't have them prior to pregnancy.

Stretch marks appear in the latter half of pregnancy on breasts and abdomen. Some women call them "love tattoos." They are red or purple to begin with. Over time they fade to white or silver and become less noticeable.

According to Mayo Clinic, there is nothing you can do to prevent stretch marks. Some women get them and others don't. It comes down to genetics. If your mother didn't have stretch marks, the likelihood is you won't either. My mom used vitamin E during her 3 pregnancies and didn't get stretch marks. (Vitamin E helps with skin elasticity.) My dermatologist recommended Mustela, which I used and didn't get marks. Though genetics count, it also makes sense to support your skin's elasticity any way you can. Complete prevention of stretch marks may not be possible, but Mustela can minimize existing stretch marks. It's also safe to use during breastfeeding.

Microderm abrasion, laser therapy and tretinoin cream are effective stretch mark treatments that can reduce visibility. Talk to your dermatologist about these after-delivery options.

Okay. How can I put this gently? One more common skin change, if you can call it that, is **hemorrhoids**. These are varicose veins in the rectum, caused by increased pressure on the uterus. Constipation adds to this uncomfortable situation. Hormones are at work again. They make your muscles and ligaments relax to make room for the baby, but they also make your intestinal muscles relax. A side-effect is that food doesn't move through the intestines as easily. Taking extra iron also causes constipation. A third factor: as pregnancy progresses, the baby presses on the bowel.

What to do: Use cold compresses, ice packs and witch hazel pads to reduce swelling. Soak in warm water. Use wet wipes instead of toilet paper. Don't sit for long periods. If you need a hemorrhoid cream, talk to your doctor about which ones are safe to use during pregnancy.

To ease constipation: Drink extra water. Eat more fiber, fruits, veggies and whole grains. Eat prunes. Drink prune juice. Get regular moderate exercise. Contact your doctor if you haven't had a bowel movement in 3 days. She will be able to recommend a stool softener safe for pregnancy.

Hair Gone Wild

It may sound weird, but your hair is part of your skin system. Increased pregnancy hormones affect hair in different ways. For many women, hair gets luxurious and thick. For others, hair goes limp, dry and even falls out (though this is usually after you give birth). Hair might also change color. Go ahead, groan. But don't worry. It will all return to normal once your hormones settle down.

Good nutrition will keep things in check. Dry brittle hair likely means you need more iron. Lack of iron is also the culprit for your new lighter shade, without a trip to the hair dresser. To maintain good hair health, eat yogurt, whole grains, almonds, cold-pressed oils, figs and dates—and take those prenatal vitamins! Give your hair a deep conditioning once a week.

Even if your locks are growing faster and thicker, hormones can make your hair as unpredictable as your mood swings. Curls can go straight, and straight can go curly. You may go to the stylist expecting a Heidi Klum-do, and come out instead looking like Andy Warhol. Get to know your new hair before making any major moves.

Easy Beauty Boosters

Nail Polish: Trend up with a vibrant new color. Be daring for under $8. Use a non-toxic nail polish (no DBP, toluene, or formaldehyde). OPI is the top non-toxic brand. If you want to splurge, get a mani pedi. You have to treat yourself every once in a while.

Color Stick: Can be used on cheeks and lips. Keeps things vibrant and your glow fresh. Blends well, especially if your skin is dry.

Concealer and Foundation: About 50% of pregnant women experience skin-tone changes. A good foundation works wonders. You may need a new shade with the right pigment for your pregnancy glow. Touch up blemishes, uneven tones or dark circles under the eyes with a concealer that is a shade or two lighter than your foundation.

Nine Ways to Feel Like a Ten

1   Wear clothes that compliment your new figure. Cleavage is there. Use it! Don't buy oversized clothing just because you have a bump.

2   Exercise. You will feel better and have more energy.

3   Get a mani-pedi. Try a new nail color.

4   Get your makeup done at a department store (it's free). Buy a new lipstick.

5   Buy a sexy nightie and undies.

6   Don't wait for a party to dress up. Do it anytime you feel like it.

7   Flirt with your husband. Meet him somewhere for a drink (just because your drink is a virgin doesn't mean you need to be one).

8   Look in the mirror and say three things you like about yourself each day.

9   What is your favorite thing to do? Go do it and have fun!

Chapter 6

I'm Never Wrong.
I'm Pregnant.

"When was the last time you were wrong?" my sister, Marisa, asked me when I was five months pregnant.

"I'm never wrong. I'm pregnant," I said. She then asked if I had noticed my increasingly irrational responses during pregnancy. "No, I haven't. I am just very particular and I want things done immediately."

"Most people would consider that irrational," Marisa said. I let her comment go, mostly to prove that she was not right about my increasing irrationality, though I suspected I *was* being irrational, but with an amnesia-like quality that made my slightly cuckoo response seem sane.

We were in the car driving through a trendy neighborhood. "Look at that astrocity," I said, about a particularly gaudy house—a big blob of white frosting and frills.

"Did you just say *astrocity?*"

I kept driving.

"That isn't a word and you say you are never wrong."

Is it wrong that I wanted to drop her off on the corner and let her walk home?

Rationality. Who needs it? Maybe your husband, to understand why you have gone round the bend several times, especially during your first trimester. The combination of mood swings and hormonal amnesia (you actually don't realize how crazy you sound, or why demanding your husband deliver a candy bar to you at 3 a.m. is out of bounds) can put even the best relationships to the test.

All your weak links will show. I believe that Nature has her biological reasons for everything. But what could be the purpose of these wild mood swings, other than scaring all would-be predators away from the growing baby?

Just because you are pregnant does not mean your relationship will get better. Instead, whatever your relationship is pre-pregnancy will be the basis for the changes to come. The huge learning curve (and curve balls) are preparing you and your partner to work as a team, smooth out your rough edges, and shape you into one unit before the baby arrives—when you'll really need strong teamwork, communication and a whole lotta love.

Mood Swings: What You Can Do

Common symptoms in the first trimester: weepy, humorless, cranky, yelling, crying and laughing at the same time, anger at nothing, and amped-up anger when there's really something to shout about, hating the smell of your own husband, craving sex, being disgusted by sex. You name it, pregnant women have felt it. Your hormones are raging, and so are you.

Emotional swings are particular to every woman, then multiplied or diminished by your partner and how he handles this shape-shifting world of pregnancy, where he sometimes feels as anxious or overwhelmed as you do, and on top of that, ignored. He secretly wonders: does he have the right as a not-so-innocent bystander without hormonal turbulence, to implode just the same? Though he's feeling that way, he'll rarely say so—especially because you might bite his head off. Some very empathetic men even take on pregnancy symptoms in the first trimester— nausea, fatigue and heightened emotional response. Talk about a double whammy! (Honey, I'm going to throw up. No, *I'm* going to throw up.)

When you feel yourself about to derail, stop and take a deep breath.

It helps to remember the stressors of new parenthood affect both partners. Particularly if it's your first child. You've been alone as a couple, used to a certain amount of normalcy and predictability, which dramatically begins to shift as soon as you get the news your family is growing. Whether planned for, hoped for, or a giant surprise—all couples go through enormous changes.

Many times, the anger issues are due to underlying fears about mortality, the health of the baby, if you're doing things right, if you'll actually be a good parent, and worries about how all these changes are affecting intimacy, domestic life, and your finances. Your husband is feeling all of these things too.

All right. That's the set up. How do you win?

Taking time for yourself on a regular basis will help mood swings. So will lots of rest, regular exercise, plenty of water (dehydration increases irritability) and frequent meals (a drop in blood sugar increases mood swings). Keep in mind that severe or lasting mood swings can indicate other problems, such as depression, which may need a doctor's attention.

Whether your symptoms include being sex-driven or suddenly developing an aversion to sex, talk about it. The way to keep your relationship going is to keep the communication flowing, and the love will too.

When you feel yourself about to derail, stop and take a deep breath. Count to ten. Try to find the humor somewhere. Anywhere. My husband and I have a code phrase: deep sleep. That's our signal for time out. A joke on those lounge-act hypnotists who can put someone into an immediate trance, no matter what is going on around them. In the middle of an argument, when one of us snaps our fingers and says, *deep sleep*, the other person has to shut their eyes and snore. It never fails to make us laugh. Try it. You can't be mad and laugh at the same time.

Mind-Body/The Biology of Stress

When you feel listened to, there is a chemical change in your body: cortisol (stress hormone) goes down. Cortisol is the culprit that causes aging, heart disease and any number of modern ills. You can control it through meditation and relaxation techniques, regular exercise, good nutrition, rest, and encouraging yourself every step of the way.

The mind-body connection is real. What we think has measurable effects on the health of our bodies. Factors for good physical, mental and emotional health include happiness, generosity, self-acceptance, gratitude, play, laughter, compassion, forgiveness—be sure to include yourself on that list.

Not only that, your baby experiences your moods too. A mother's overall emotional state affects her baby's emotional state. Stressed mothers tend to deliver stressed babies. Mothers who are supported by their partners during pregnancy have less stressful births, with fewer problems during delivery.

It makes sense for you and your partner to get a handle on stress and understand there are delightful solutions, such as doing things you enjoy and deeply supporting one another in your new role as parents. Here are some tips on making that happen:

- Your partner won't be able to give everything you need. Accept your partner as he is and yourself too. In a moment of sanity, talk about your mood swings. Clue him in, so that he'll be able to help instead of feeling helpless.

- Develop relationships outside your relationship. Mommy groups, friends, social networks, supportive family, church, community, to name a few solid resources.

- Don't ignore your own needs. Know when to give and when you need to receive. Don't feel embarrassed by asking for help or advice. Just talking to a sympathetic friend can often alleviate stress and give you new ideas to your present impasse.

- Listen, empathize. When you have time together with your husband, talk about your shared hopes for the future, not what is left to do, or who hasn't done what… Let your partner know you believe in him, and vice versa—you need to hear his confidence in you. Compliment yourselves as a couple.

Raising the Love Meter: Stay Physical

Be inventive in your love life—even if you have none. Stay physical. Oxytocin (also known as the love hormone, crucial to bonding) is released just by touching the lips or cuddling, as well as during sex. If you're feeling sexless, you can still dance, cuddle, listen, laugh, and talk about your love. Say what you admire about each other. Remember how grateful you are for his patience, or whatever qualities you treasure in your partner. It can't be fake just to keep the peace. Gratitude in relationships is an actual psychological factor for long-term success.

And more than anything, you both are hoping for long-term success in your new family dynamics as Mom and Dad.

Write down what you love, what you dream of. Try to think past the current craziness and remember you have a life to live, and dreams of your own, and a partner to share them with. Be sure that as a couple, you don't limit your conversation only to baby talk (though that's easy to do with so many pressures and changes).

Date Night

- Entertain Me: There's nothing like theater, good music or a dance concert to swoop you away to another time and place. Movies are a great option as well.

- Mama Hungry: Dinner out with your partner is always a winner—especially when you are eating for two!

- Too Tired to Go Out? Have a mocktail party. Invite friends over for good food & conversation. You could even play a few rounds of your favorite game. Charades anyone?

  * My Favorite Mocktails: Cranberry juice and sparkling water spritzer. Pomegranate-apple rossini: 1 part pomegranate juice to 5 parts chilled sparkling apple cider. Serve in champagne flute. Add lemon twist.

Babymoons

Babymoons are a great way to reconnect with your partner, and refresh yourselves before the baby is born. Most couples schedule their babymoon in the third trimester. By then you'll have settled most of the delivery planning, made headway on collecting your baby essentials, and no doubt could use a good vacation.

- Choose some place you will both enjoy, and not so far away that it will take an exhausting 3 days to get there.

- Stay within your budget. Finances become a larger concern as delivery time nears.

- Even if it's a weekend, a night away, or just a few days of playful staycation, never underestimate the rejuvenating effects of play, fun, and laughter.

Single Moms

There are nearly 14 million single parents in the U.S. today, most of them single moms. Every mom needs loving support, good advice, and access to resources. The biggest issue for single moms is the overload of trying to do everything yourself, or feeling you must go it alone. Healthy pregnancy and emotional support go hand-in-hand. Trusted friends, family, and a good doctor/healthcare professional make a great team.

Take the time to set up your support system. Connect with other moms in your area. Use Internet social networks and community resources.

Ask for help when you need it.

Though you are busy, make time for fun. Schedule play dates for yourself and your girlfriends/guyfriends. It is a proven medical fact that friends are good for your health. Nurturing friendships lower stress, boost the immune system and lengthen lifespan.

Feel like you need more support or just want to connect with other mommies? Most communities have Mommy Groups or free parenting classes. Can't find one? Create one! Start by asking the moms you know if they would be interested, and start a weekly or monthly get together. You can also Google online communities or become a member of your favorite mommy website. Most mommy websites allow you to post comments and get advice.

There are many single parenting websites. One of the best is www.singlemothers.org.

Chapter 7

Getting Ready Physically
and Emotionally

Bonding Begins in the Womb

Think your baby is just hanging out in your uterus, swimming around, waiting to be delivered? Think again. In the womb, babies dream, have memories and suck their thumbs. Consider these amazing facts:

- A pregnant woman's voice reverberates through her body. Babies prefer their own mother's voice and recognize it immediately–even in a birth-room full of people.

- In the womb, babies are learning about language. From the moment of birth, infants cry in the accent of their mother's native tongue.

- Babies whose mothers read *The Cat in the Hat* to them while pregnant, recognized passages from the book.

- Babies of women who watched a certain soap opera every day while pregnant, recognized the theme song.

Nine months is a long time. Your baby is busy soaking in not just nutrients, but the emotional environment that surrounds his mother. Sounds, air, water, mood, food—your baby is absorbing it all, and using the information to calculate what to expect from life.

At 23 weeks, your baby has a sense of movement and can feel you dance! She can also hear, so put on some music and sway. At 28 weeks, the taste and smell are fully developed. After birth, infants prefer the foods their mothers ate during pregnancy, including spices. They also prefer their mother's smell over all others. Though playing Mozart will not make your baby a genius, if the music soothes you, it will likely soothe him too.

Babies prefer their own mother's voice. Read and sing to your baby, laugh and talk with her.

Read to your little love bug, sing to her, laugh and talk. She's there and she's listening, and already loves the sound of your voice.

Designing the Nursery: Setting Up Serenity

The nesting instinct is an actual physical symptom of pregnancy. It can begin anywhere from mid-term to a few weeks before delivery. You'll recognize it by your crazed desire to scrub every nook and cranny, organize all the closets in your house, and color-code your baby's wardrobe. For most women, designing the nursery is a lot of fun. You may be creating a nest in a corner of your bedroom, or have a larger space to work with. No matter how big or small your space or budget, the overall design should be both practical and inspiring.

Color: If you plan on having more than one child, choose a gender-neutral wall color. It's a temptation to do bright, primary colors, but these can excite the baby. Restful pastels are best. Try green, blue, pale yellow, or ivory. Paint the room at least two months before the baby is due. Keep room ventilated to release toxic fumes. Eco-friendly paints like milk- and clay-based formulas work beautifully too. They need one month airing time.

Theme: Add a fun mural to the wall. I found a self-adhesive jungle-theme mural at Target for under $20. Easy to apply and makes the room joyful.

Think through the logistics: Does it make sense to have onesies in the closet or in the drawer of the changing table? Since you don't want to leave your baby unattended on the table, it's helpful to have all changing necessities within arm's reach, including a soft light for night changes. You may want a small table beside your feeding chair (rockers are great) for anything you might need—water, mommy snacks, burp cloths, pacifier, timer.

Babies grow so fast, there's no need to invest in top-of-the-line for everything. Borrow where you can. Your mom friends will likely have newborn items their babies have outgrown. My sister-in-law lent me a great changing table. If you borrow a baby crib, make sure it meets current safety standards.

Create room for adaptability: You'll be tempted to make the nursery all about baby, but consider your own needs too. For my last trimester, I arranged to work part-time at home and part-time at the office. I created a small work station in the nursery—a tabletop attached to the wall to save space. As babies are so sensitive, it's best to keep electronics and wireless devices away from the crib. My preference is the all-natural nursery with as few gadgets as possible.

The nursery layout will likely change once the baby arrives, and you actually begin to use the space.

Guiding Principles

As I decorated the nursery with books and art that reflected who I wanted my child to be, I thought about what I valued in life and the core beliefs I hoped to instill in my children. I ended up writing four core principles—gentle reminders of the ideals that would help guide our children through life's twists and turns.

They have become my family's guiding principles, printed and framed in each one of our rooms.

Or make your own guiding principles. Get your husband involved in the project. Dream together. Give thought to what you care about most, and what traits you want your children to carry on from your life experiences. From time to time, we all need reminders about how we should treat others and what our driving force should be.

- Do what makes you **happy**, makes you smile and feel alive. Let happiness guide the decisions you make in life, so long as that happiness is balanced with responsibility.

- **Love** freely and with all your heart. Don't be afraid to give or receive love, for it is one of the most precious gifts we can experience. Love yourself—focus on your strengths, not your faults.

- **Respect and be kind** to yourself and to others. Treat others as you want to be treated. Every person experiences life in a different way; try to understand and have compassion for their point of view.

- **Education** will expand your opportunities and choices in life—take it seriously.

Nursery Essentials

Good nursery design keeps baby *&* mom in mind.
A haven for you both. A place to have fun with your
little one, while being so peaceful that your baby
will be sleeping through the night in no time!

☐ **Crib & Mattress** $
- Slats do not exceed 2 3/8"
- No drop-side frames
- Converts into toddler bed. Saves $ in the long run.
- Organic mattress; or use BabeSafe cover on standard mattress.

☐ **Glider/Rocking Chair** $
- Big enough to fit you, your baby & your breastfeeding pillow.
- Use a small stool as a footrest vs. spending more on an ottoman.

☐ **Monitor**
- Video & audio capabilities
- Low interference/multichannel
- Portable receiver(s): plug-in or battery. Choose long battery life & good range.

☐ **Changing Table**
- Table with shelves or drawers for storage
- Easy-to-clean changing pad
- 2-3 washable pad covers

☐ **Diaper Trashcan**
- Easy to open, with lid
- Step & drop design

☐ **Swing**
- Various speeds, plays music
- Safety harness
- For newborns, a reclining seat is best until they have neck control.

☐ **Stationary Exersaucer**
- Adjustable height positions to grow with your baby
- Machine washable seat cover

☐ **Play Mat for Tummy Time**
- Start at 2 weeks old to strengthen baby's back, neck & spine.
- Mat should be compact, easy to move, with few loose parts.

☐ **Books**
- Fairytales, art, poems, stories, nature, humor. Books of all kinds.
- Read to your child every day. Bedtime stories are fun & act as a signal for baby to wind-down & sleep.

☐ **Toys**
- Easy to catch & hold ball
- Interactive musical toy
- Stuffed animals to cuddle

$ = Money Saver

Chapter 8

Practical Matters

Maternity Leave

Paid maternity leave is normal in most countries (for moms *and* dads), except for the United States. We are the only industrialized country in the world that does not offer paid maternity leave. What's on offer in our country is 12-weeks of job-protected, unpaid leave. But the federal laws apply only to larger companies of 50 or more employees, which means most working moms don't have job protection if they take time off with their babies. This needs to change!

Studies show that women who take maternity leave have healthier babies and stronger families. Three months is ideal, but the average leave time in the U.S. is 10.5 weeks, with many moms unable to take that much time off work. Whatever your situation, do your best to plan ahead and take full advantage of the resources available.

Some smart, compassionate companies have their own paid maternity-leave policy. California and New Jersey have paid family leave programs. Hawaii, New York and Rhode Island have short-term disability insurance programs that cover a portion of a woman's wages during maternity leave. Other ways to buy time: trade in vacation, sick leave, or family days.

Check out all your options. Make sure to do any required paperwork early in your pregnancy, so you can plan your budget and time effectively. Once you have all the information, sit down with your partner and decide how much leave-time you can financially afford.

Many states and employers offer voluntary short-term disability plans you can pay into, that help cover wage loss during maternity leave. Contact the Human Resources Department at your workplace to find out exactly what choices are available to you.

If your boss and work are flexible, arrange to work part-time from your home in the last trimester. The flexible work schedule allows you to get the rest you need to prepare for delivery, while devoting most of your maternity leave where you'll need it most: postpartum recovery and adjusting to the new life in your life.

If flexibility is not an option, do your best to plan a lighter, more manageable workload as you near delivery. Talk with co-workers who have had babies and ask for practical tips on work and leave. Inform your employer early on about the amount of leave time you plan to take and when. The Family Leave law requires a 30-day notice for unpaid maternity leave. Be proactive. Discuss details with your employer, such as who might be best to cover your workload, project concerns, and suggestions for a smooth transition.

Budget Boosters

- Sort through old clothes or items that you no longer use. Post them on eBay or Craigslist, have a garage sale, or use a consignment store. Clearing out your home will create fresh new space, as well as generating some cash.

- Sign up for a credit card that gives you cash back for purchases. Put the cash back bonus into your savings or toward credit card payments. If possible, pay off the card at the end of each month to avoid interest charges.

- You'll need to cut back anyway on caffeine. Put the money you would have spent at a coffee shop into savings.

- Bring your lunch to work. It will be healthier and a lot less expensive. If you want to get out of the office, find a park or patio nearby and have a picnic.

- Go over your monthly bills and see where you can streamline. For instance, cut back on your cable bill; avoid overcharges on your cell phone plan for extra minutes; if you don't use your landline much, consider disconnecting it.

- Bottle your own water. Buy a stainless steel water bottle and refill it at home or work. A 20 oz. bottle of water costs $1.50. Multiply that by the 3+ bottles a day you need during pregnancy. You could save roughly $1,200 over nine months.

- Don't be shy about telling friends you are on a baby budget. When it's time for girls' night out, cheap and cheerful can be just as fun as more expensive eateries.

Chapter 9

Preparing for Delivery

Choosing Your Doctor

From the start of your first trimester onward, prenatal care is important. Making an appointment with your doctor or midwife is one of the first things you should do. Choosing a provider is a personal matter. If you feel your current doctor will not suit your pregnancy needs, interview others until you find a healthcare professional you are comfortable with. Some women feel better with a crisp, no-nonsense doctor, while others need a more emotional connection. There is no right or wrong. This decision is about you, your choices and comfort levels.

Ask questions. Check out your potential provider's professional standing, how long they've been in practice, what hospitals/clinics they work through, and who are their back-up practitioners. It's important their approach aligns with your birthing desires. Do they routinely use intervention during labor? Do they work with doulas? Support natural childbirth decisions? What is their stance on C-sections, amniocentesis? What tests do they recommend and why? If you have any special needs, be up front about it. A good doctor will be willing to give thorough answers and make sure you understand your options.

I wanted a doctor who was willing to take time with me, and take even my perhaps silly questions seriously. I interviewed several ob-gyns. The first two didn't cut it. One lived too far away. The other tried to cut me short when I needed answers. The third was a charm.

Professional, supportive, a good listener who had the kind of thorough answers and open approach that made me feel I could trust my body and my baby in her hands.

Choosing a Birth Plan

Birth plans are a useful tool to help you ask the right questions in advance, and to make sure you, your husband, and your doctor are in agreement about your informed consent on a number of important issues concerning delivery. Make the decisions together. Include your partner in as many planning activities as possible. New dads are as unsure as new moms. Getting involved at the planning stage helps him better understand his role and feel confident about it.

Work with your doctor and partner to create the birth you want.

If you are a single mom, choose a trusted friend or family member to be your birthing partner and accompany you through all the stages.

How detailed you get with your birth plan is up to you, but the important issues for me were:

- What kind of environment you want during labor (who's in the room, can they take photographs, do you want music?).

- What kind of pain relief you want during labor and after delivery. Options range from natural methods such as acupressure, to epidural. If you are having a C-section, after-delivery pain relief is an important choice.

- Do you want to immediately hold your baby once delivered, or have him/her washed and swaddled first?

- Which baby medical exams you approve, and whether you prefer they be done in your presence.

- Feeding info for nursing team: breast milk only or formula? Schedule or feed-on-demand? Are pacifiers okay?

- Circumcision: yes or no?

Educate Yourself

"Am I ready for this?" every pregnant woman asks herself, especially as her pregnancy progresses and things become REAL. The physical changes begin to bear down on you. The weight of the baby is shifting your pelvis, your belly keeps bumping into doors and strangers, incontinence is your new worst friend. Laughing is good for you, but you're afraid to laugh for fear of dribbling—even with those 50 Kegels a day!

"Am I ready for this?" Very often our answer is No! I'm terrified, overwhelmed and don't like pain. What if something goes wrong, and which "wrong" would it be? There are so many possibilities! What if, what if, and then? Anxiety is normal, but that doesn't make you less anxious. Your husband, too, is feeling the pressure.

Everyone has different measures of what makes them feel ready. Other mothers are a great resource. Ask as many as you can about everything. "Ready" for me meant reading every book I could get my hands on about pregnancy, delivery, and motherhood—until I was so overwhelmed, I couldn't remember anything. I took copious notes, but when I later tried to make sense of them, I felt like the Blob had eaten my homework. There is a balance between being informed and being obsessed.

My delivering hospital, Cedars-Sinai, offered a variety of classes. Drawing on their expertise, I was better able to process the information I needed, as well as ask questions that weren't necessarily in the books I had read. I also liked meeting other new parents, and seeing we all shared the same anxious, elated confusion and euphoria. Most delivering hospitals offer classes to new parents. The following are the classes I took which were most beneficial to me:

- **Prepared Childbirth:** Taught by an experienced nurse, Adriano and I learned about pregnancy, delivery, breastfeeding and what to expect the first few weeks of parenthood. The class included hands-on teamwork for both partners, practicing delivery exercises and breathing techniques for a rewarding birth experience.

- **Breastfeeding:** I took a class specifically on breastfeeding since my goal was to breastfeed for at least the first 6 months.

- **Child Safety:** Adriano and I learned infant CPR and general safety guidelines for our home and garden areas.

Practical Preparations

I also recommend taking a tour of your delivering hospital prior to birth, so you and your partner know your way around the place, especially admissions, maternity ward and delivery area. Be sure all your insurance paperwork is done in advance. While you're in labor, the last place you want to be is stuck at reception reading the fine print.

Have a Plan A for Awesome in place (everything goes perfectly as expected) and Plan B for But What If? (my husband/birth partner isn't available when I go into labor, my water breaks early...). Plan B should include a trusted back-up to drive you to the hospital (do NOT drive yourself!), and a printout of what you plan to take to the hospital, in case you need a friend to pack your things for you. (See page 74, *What You Will Need at the Hospital.*) If you have other children at home, a trusted childcare helper on call during your last trimester is a must.

Chapter 10

Birthing Options

My Father was a Doula

As a new mother, you're going to get advice, much of it conflicting. My mother was a natural woman. You know, the 70s kind, with long flowing hair, who ate whole grains way back when, with a kitchen full of honey, homemade yogurt and fresh baked bread. A natural woman in favor of natural childbirth. At home. On her own bed. No drugs, no doctors or *episiotomies*. Just a deep trust in the wisdom of her body, and a deep trust in my father—who was her doula. My father had actually assisted in a number of births, he was so good at making new moms feel at ease. He had a beautiful singing voice and used it to create calm in the delivery room. This is true. How could I make this stuff up? My parents had three children, all by natural childbirth.

I was delivered by my own father, whose voice and loving support could soothe the gnarliest labor pains. *Breathe breathe breathe.* My parents used the Lamaze method and it worked for them. My sister and brother were delivered by midwives. My sister, at home. My brother at a small Red Cross clinic. Every birth was a perfect one. Not a stitch or a tear. It goes to show that birthing is easier if you have that kind of trust. But having that kind of trust, at least for me, is hard.

My mother-in-law, on the other hand, is a princess. Susan birthed in a state-of-the-art hospital in Rome, and used an epidural. Her advice to me: "Take the pain killers! You're going to need them."

You will have to choose what is both practical and meaningful for you. Natural childbirth, water-birthing, or traditional Western? At home, birthing center, hospital—or a birthing center in a hospital? Midwife or ob-gyn? Self-hypnosis pain techniques, mild pain blockers or full epidural? The good news is each woman can choose the type of birth that meets her emotional and physical needs, depending upon your health and what is available in your local area. Birth is about empowerment—getting to know your body intimately, confronting your fears and understanding what *you* want in terms of delivery. Both surrender and taking charge.

My friend, Jennifer, chose to deliver her twins vaginally, instead of the routinely recommended C-section. Another friend, Dante, chose water birth at home with a midwife—in part because she didn't have insurance, but also because she's drawn to natural practices, as well as the idea that water birth is less painful because the water takes pressure off your uterus and the baby. My friend, Missy, liked the comfort of full hospital attendance and the painkillers that went with it. They all had successful births and were happy with their choices.

I wanted my childbirth to be as natural as possible, while being in the safest environment possible. So I chose natural childbirth (meaning drug-free with minimal medical intervention) in a good hospital and found an excellent ob-gyn. I also hired Amy, an experienced doula recommended by a friend.

During my last trimester, I met with Amy weekly to prepare myself both emotionally and physically for natural childbirth. A doula is not a midwife. She is more like a personal trainer for childbirth. She provides continuous physical, emotional and informational support to the mother before, during, and just after childbirth. A nurturing presence for both mother and father in helping them cope with labor.

"Women who are birthing in a hospital need two kinds of knowing," Amy explained. "The primordial knowing; that innate capability which modern women have, but must rediscover and trust. The second is modern knowing, being savvy about the medical and hospital culture and how to give birth within it. In birth preparation your first task is to empty your mind of expectations and judgments that narrow the possibilities of coping with pain, surprises, and the hard work of labor."

In other words, instinct isn't instinctual anymore. We've been educated away from trusting what our bodies know. A big part of my birth training was understanding how to relax and let my body do the work. That meant dropping stress, fear, and worry. But how?

Tackling the Worry Factor

Worry is an illusion. Most of your fears never happen. But your body doesn't know it. When you worry, you tend to go over a troubling thought hundreds of times a day. (The average person has a whopping 50,000 thoughts per day. For men, half of those are about sex!) Your brain tells your body, and your body reacts as if that worry is actually happening. It releases stress hormones and you go into fight-or-flight response.

Most of our worries never happen. Focusing on positive outcomes creates better results.

The opposite is also true. By imagining good results, focusing on happy desirable thoughts, you project trust into your future. Your brain tells your body all is well and you relax, which actually brings you closer to really having the happy outcomes you want. The more sensory detail you use in your imagining (smell, taste, touch, how good it feels to achieve your goal), the more real your brain and body take it as an actual physical experience.

In a famous study, two basketball teams were in training. One practiced on the court an extra hour a day. The other spent that hour in pure visualization, imagining the perfect shots, the victory, the moves they made to do it. Guess which team actually improved the most? The visualizers. Top athletes from Olympic gold medalists to NBA teams to golf champions regularly use visualization to improve their game.

You can use it, too, because birthing is a marathon. The physical equivalent of running five miles in a flat-out sprint. In their pregnancy handbook, *Prepared Childbirth—the Family Way*, authors Debby Amis and Jeanne Green suggest using relaxation techniques (mental imagery) and some of the following positive affirmations in preparing for delivery:

- Every day my baby grows stronger.

- I feel calm and at peace with the world.

- My baby gives me strength to labor.

- My body is made to give birth.

- I am strong and able to birth my baby.

Pick one or two that feel right to you and say them whenever you find yourself fretting about delivery. You can't just do them once in a while. Make it a daily practice, as beneficial to your body as those delivery exercises you've been doing. The more you do it, the easier it gets.

Fear of Pain and How to Handle It

In addition to weekly doula meetings, I worked on hypnobirthing techniques an hour a day after work. Hypnobirthing is a form of self-hypnosis to talk yourself out of fear. It's not the pain, but the fear of pain during labor that causes the worst discomfort. Remember:

- Your body knows what to do, if only you will let it.

- Educate yourself about what is happening during childbirth, so that fear is diminished and your body can do its job more effectively.

- Know the patterns of labor, the length of contractions and quiet space in between, the increased pacing that signals you are about to succeed in a miracle: birth.

- Ride the waves of labor through controlled breathing and meditative exercises such as focusing on a serene mental image (mine was Lake Como in Italy).

- Don't be afraid of the pain. Learn to release it and focus on your amazing body doing its beautiful work.

Yes, these were the things I learned from my doula and daily practice of hypnobirthing relaxation tapes. I was ready.

Chapter 11

Signs of Labor

It looks easy in the movies. The pregnant woman is standing in a sudden gush of water, as unmistakable as Niagara Falls. Or she is gripped by a contraction so body-bending that all she can do is scream, "Quick! It's time!"

Reality: sometimes your water can break in a small trickle, and all you think is, "When is this #?!&%*! incontinence going to end!?" Or you get excited as you feel contractions begin, then find out they are just Braxton Hicks contractions, otherwise known as false labor. Your uterus's dress rehearsal, practicing up for the real thing. Braxton Hicks contractions are common in the last trimester. False labor can sometimes be painful, or simply feel like an odd tightening in the abdomen.

Only 1 in 10 women experience the gush when water breaks.

Every woman is different. Though there are no hard and fast rules about how your body is going to behave as delivery time nears, you can learn a few simple signals that will help you tell the difference between false labor and real labor.

Quick & Easy: False vs. True Labor

1 Time the contractions (when they start and when they stop, and also the interval between). Real labor pains have a regular pattern, and continue to grow stronger and closer together. False labor is irregular and the pain level is generally weaker than true contractions.

2 Real contractions last over 30 seconds in the beginning, and stretch to 70-90 seconds long as labor progresses. False contractions have irregular patterns of length and progression.

3 If you are really in labor, there is nothing you can do to stop it. Whether you are walking or lying down, the pains will keep coming like a train right on schedule. With false labor, you may be able to control the pains by varying activities or position.

4 Early true labor can feel like menstrual cramps, and are initially felt as dull lower back pain which moves forward into the abdomen. You will also feel pressure on the pelvis and possibly the need to urinate. False contractions tend to be felt in the front of the abdomen.

Preterm labor: call your doctor if you have signs of early labor (before 36 weeks) – especially if you see vaginal spotting.

Signals Delivery Time is Near

Lightening: The baby lowers from under the ribcage into your pelvis in preparation for delivery. For first-time moms, lightening occurs anywhere from a few hours to a few weeks before delivery. (With subsequent babies, the drop usually happens during delivery.) Some women notice the signs, while others do not. You may be able to breathe easier, as your ribcage is better able to expand. But the uterus is also putting more pressure on the bladder and rectum. In some women, this results in an increased need to urinate (yes, even more than you already do) or you may feel the baby could drop right out of you. Don't worry—it won't!

Passing the mucous plug: otherwise known as the "bloody show." Who knew your cervix had a plug? Throughout your pregnancy, the mucous plug has been blocking the opening to your cervix so bacteria cannot enter the uterus. As birthing time nears, your cervix begins to open and the plug is released. This can occur anywhere from a few hours to several weeks away from delivery. The mucous plug will appear as a thick, clear or pink discharge from the vagina.

Water breaking: Forget what you've seen in the movies. Only one in ten women experience the gush. And water most commonly breaks during labor, not before. Normally once your water breaks, it's a signal that delivery will be soon. Technically, water breaking is the rupture of the amniotic membrane. The amniotic fluid may pour out in a gush or a slow steady trickle. The fluid is clear (or hay-color) and odorless—it's what your baby has been swimming in the past 9 months.

Sometimes it's not easy to tell between incontinence and water breaking. If you are not sure, examine the odor and color. Amniotic fluid does not smell like urine. Water breaking will usually soak a panty liner, and may continue to leak. If you can't determine which one it is, contact your healthcare professional or make an office visit.

When the real thing happens, write down the time your water breaks, the amount of fluid (gush or trickle, intermittent or continued), its color and odor, then call your doctor.

- If you are in labor and the sac has not broken, it will usually happen sometime during labor. If not, your doctor will rupture the membrane—a safe and painless procedure.

- Don't worry if your water breaks before you go into labor (premature rupture of the membrane). For most women, labor follows soon after. Notify your doctor.

- If your water breaks before 37 weeks, call your doctor and follow all instructions.

The Three Stages of Labor

Stage 1: Early Labor and Active Labor

This the longest stage, and is divided into two parts.

Early Labor: For first-time moms, early labor can last from several hours to several days. (With subsequent births, it's usually quicker.) Contractions may be mild to moderately strong as your cervix dilates (begins to open for birth). It's a good time for gentle distractions and relaxing activities. Go for a walk or take a warm shower, watch a movie, listen to music. If you're hungry, eat lightly. Drink plenty of fluids. If you are feeling lower back pain, use a hot compress or ice pack. If it is night, try to sleep. Conserve your energy for birthing.

Keep track of your contractions (the length and intervals between). Get your spouse or birthing partner to help you time them. In the early labor phase, contractions generally begin 15 to 20 minutes apart, and can last from 30 to 90 seconds.

Active Labor: Contractions get longer, stronger, and closer in intervals. When contractions quicken to less than 5 minutes apart, it is time to go to the hospital. Work with your birthing team. Keep breathing. Stay focused. Ask for what you need—whether pain relief, a gentle massage between contractions, cold compresses on your forehead, a warm shower or a walk down the hall. Rocking helps. Relax as much as possible, even if the pains are so close together, you feel like you are riding one giant tsunami wave. During active labor, your cervix dilates to 10 centimeters to allow the baby to pass through.

The last part of active labor is called the transition. You may feel the need to push, but unless you are fully dilated, your doctor or midwife will ask you to hold back. Pushing when you're not fully dilated can cause tearing. According to my mom, natural childbirth Olympian, this is the time when focus counts, but it's also the time when you really want to scream. It's the most difficult phase of labor, but happily also the shortest—from ½ hour to 1 ½ hours.

Stage 2: Birth

Okay, go ahead and push. You are fully dilated. It's show time! Now is the time to actively work with your contractions. This part of the delivery can take a few minutes to a few hours. Each birth is different. If you've birthed before, pushing the baby through often comes easily. If you're a first-time mom, or if you've had an epidural, you'll likely need more time to allow the vaginal opening to stretch to adequate size, so there is no tearing.

Your doctor or midwife will guide you through the process, which can be gentle (waiting to push until you feel the urge) or accelerated (pushing with each contraction). Out-of-bed positions are becoming more popular. Water pools, birthing stools, birth chairs and birth balls are a few of the options that may make the big push easier. Squatting opens the pelvis by ten percent.

When you push, remember to bear down in the lower part of your body. Here is where your months of muscle-isolating delivery exercises come in handy. Don't allow tension to gather in your facial muscles. Direct your energies to the task at hand—pushing your baby into the world. Once your baby's head is delivered, the body follows easily.

Stage 3: Delivery of the Placenta

This is the shortest stage, lasting about ten minutes to half-an-hour. One last push for the placenta to be delivered, and you're home free. You'll still be having mild contractions, but these are nothing compared to what you have just been through and the triumph you will feel as you hold your baby for the first time.

Chapter 12

Here He Comes!

At 35 weeks my baby flipped feet-first. I tried acupuncture, hoping for another flip that would set him into proper birthing position, but he was too big and it was too late to make that sort of move.

I felt a failure somehow. The natural delivery I had envisioned was not going to happen. No doula. No hypnobirthing. All the training I had worked on so hard was for nothing. Breech. C-section. Everything out of my control. After more than a few good cries, I tried to get some perspective.

Cesarean delivery is now the most common surgical procedure in US hospitals. More than 1.2 million births a year. But it is still major abdominal surgery. Vaginal delivery is preferable in most cases, as the risk of complication and recovery time (for mom and baby) are lower. Nonetheless, for a 30+ mom like me whose baby decided to go breech, it's the healthiest, lowest-risk option.

So I wouldn't be able to use my natural birthing techniques for the birth itself, but my daily practice of relaxation hypnosis and meditation had prepared me to accept gracefully this new turn of events, so to speak. Already motherhood was teaching me a few things about letting go. Who knows? Maybe the baby knew better than I. Maybe he was breech for a reason. I twirled the downside into up, cheering myself on as I scheduled the C-section, and then realized, quite happily, I could choose my baby's birthday: 09/09/09. Why not have fun with this?

What You Will Need at the Hospital

You want to feel as comfortable as possible in the hospital. As you pack your suitcase, think of the things that bring you comfort. Here's what I took with me:

- ☐ My own pillow and pajamas

- ☐ Nursing pillow

- ☐ Warm socks and slippers

- ☐ A warm scarf in case the room is too cold; a hand fan if the room is too hot

- ☐ Nutritious snacks—don't rely on hospital food

- ☐ Underwear. If you are having a C-section, bring panties large enough to avoid any pressure around the C-section incision. Low-rise cut doesn't work because the elastic will be touching the incision area.

- ☐ Nursing bras and nipple relief pads. Ameda ComfortGel Hydrogel Pads work best.

- ☐ Comfortable feminine pads

- ☐ Toiletries (deodorant, razor, toothbrush, toothpaste, etc.)

- ☐ Makeup (photos please!) and lip balm

- ☐ Camera and/or video camera

- ☐ My iPhone which had a soothing music playlist

- ☐ Electronics charger

- ☐ Mom's and baby's outfits to wear home

Ready or Not...

I was prepared for everything, except the panic that overtook me as my doctor sat me up on the delivery table, and told me to hunch over so staff could put the needle into my spine. I tried to forget what I knew about possible complications, tried to blank out—where was my husband? He wasn't allowed in yet, the delivery room was freezing, blue blank lights, my mother somewhere in the hospital. Where had I left her?

Adriano suddenly, almost magically, appeared at my side. I heard his far-away voice, bubbling from somewhere inside his blue surgical shower cap, telling me everything was going to be okay—though even in my drug-fog, I could see a similar panic in his eyes. The delivery staff turned on the radio. A song came on my dad used to sing to me when we were far away from each other: *somewhere out there, someone's saying a prayer, someone's thinking of you....loving you...* I started to cry uncontrollably. Then a soft peace settled in and I seemed to be watching it all in third person.

At exactly 1:00 p.m. on 09/09/09, Alessio was born. He weighed in at 8 pounds, 4 ounces, and 21 inches long. So big, the doctor wasn't sure she could deliver him through a normal-sized incision, but she managed. I winced at the thought of tiny me trying to naturally deliver a baby whose head-size measured in the 98th percentile. I was thankful Alessio had the good sense to go breech.

He was beautiful, of course, as every mother will say as she first lays eyes on her newborn. Even if he did look like a little Yoda. An old man in a 21-inch body, staring up at me with a sense of contemplation, an odd little skew of dismay in his eyes as he gazed around the room, that he was here in this world, this bright cold world full of lights and noises and no water to swim in, only his swaddling that made him feel safe. Then my voice. He knew it from the womb. I could see him relax as I talked to him, settle into my arms with a sense of peace.

I kept listening, watching his scrunched up little face for clues on how to communicate, what he was feeling, how to know what I should know, but didn't yet. I was only beginning to sense the enormity and wonder of what lay ahead.

After a few elated moments holding my baby, he was whisked away. Alessio had low body temperature. My husband followed the nurses and baby somewhere into the hospital labyrinth where monitoring and testing would be done, while I was being monitored in the post-op recovery room. I was shivering uncontrollably. I'd never been so cold. I had read about shaking being a possible side-effect of an epidural, but nobody mentioned this fierce, rattle-your-teeth shivering. That, combined with worries about my baby's health, made the first hour after delivery an excruciating fog of unknowing, where it seemed the only thing I could say was: "Where is my baby? Is he all right?"

The fuzzy warm euphoria I had imagined—the three of us together oohing and ahhing, the celebratory procession wheeling down the hallway holding my baby—was instead a time of anxiety. It's a strange thing, after all the fanfare of birth, that new moms can get placed on the backburner, as far as information relay goes. It was the longest, loneliest hour of my life.

The euphoria came about an hour later when Papa and baby returned with the news all was well. Nothing was wrong with Alessio's body temperature. The thermometer had been broken!

My hard-won advice: don't worry until somebody tells you it's time to worry, which hopefully will not come. Even if there are health concerns with your newborn, a good team of doctors will help you through it all. New mom terrors are common. Understand it's okay to cry, blubber or shiver to the bones. Scream if you want. You've been through a lot. But you'll only realize it later, looking back, that nothing can adequately prepare you for the enormous emotional and physical feat of giving birth.

Take advantage of your hospital's team of experts, available at the push of a button.

I spent the next three days in the hospital. Since cesarean is considered major surgery, a longer hospital stay is required—48 to 72 hours, as opposed to the typical 24-48 hours for a vaginal delivery.

I was grateful to have a nurse by my side who reassured me that all Alessio's reactions and fusses were "normal, nothing to worry about, just do this or that, a swaddle here, a burp there. Sing to him, hold him, pat him on your chest, hold him this way, not that—oh let him find his own way—he will tell you," she said.

Take advantage of your hospital's team of experts, available at the push of a button—bedside or in the bathroom, 24/7. This is a luxury that allows you to get the deep rest you need, both in recovering from birth and preparing for the next big step—home alone with baby!

Second Time Around

The second time around (1½ years later), I had a C-section, but shivering was expected and thermometer was working. I held my newborn for a good long time and was able to nurse while in the recovery room. We had our little family parade, as Adriano and the nurse wheeled Sienna and me to our room, where the four of us oohed and aahed—Alessio was there waiting to welcome his sister into the world.

What a difference in post-birth experiences. I am grateful for both, for what each taught me. Having to face your fears when things go wrong makes you a lot stronger. The second-time around I had more courage and was less afraid. I had less expectations for "the perfect birth" and greater confidence that I could handle whatever came.

Perfect Birth? What's That?

I think most moms' desires for a "perfect birth" have to do with fear of the unknown. The lack of control we feel when our water breaks, contractions begin, and we have to deliver ourselves into the hands of the experts while our bodies take over. Whether you birth vaginally or by C-section, birthing takes a huge amount of trust. You simply have to let go and surrender to the experience.

My friend Jennifer's first babies were twins. She wanted to deliver both vaginally, though her doctor recommended the normal C-section delivery for twins. Jennifer got her way in the end, with a few unexpected twists. In her own words:

"When it came time to start pushing for Christian, Baby A, the nurse told me to push as hard as I could while she counted to ten. I didn't realize how hard I was pushing because my husband, Tom, said urine came out of me like a hose, so hard that it knocked the doctor back and sprayed all over his face. This happened twice, one right after the other, until they finally put a catheter in me. The doctor was NOT happy with that nurse. I was so humiliated the next day, knowing I had given my doctor a 'golden shower!' It took a long time to push Christian out. When I finally did, I felt so relieved it was over, I forgot I had another one to push out. Ethan came just six minutes later. Two pushes, then I was finally done.

"Going through the whole journey of my pregnancy with three months of bed rest, almost pre-term labor at 27 weeks, and the birthing process gave me such a sense of accomplishment. I still had a lot of fear. There was still a huge sense of the unknown, bringing home two babies and having to raise them. But I felt empowered, too, knowing that I did my best."

What to Expect Postpartum at the Hospital

- Breastfeed the baby as soon as you are able, within the first hour if possible.

- The nurse will get you up and walking as soon as possible, which will speed your recovery. You'll need help, and thankfully, help is what you've got 24/7.

- Every few hours, nurses will check your body temperature, incision (cesarean) or stitches (episiotomy), vaginal blood flow, pain medication and make any adjustments necessary. Vaginal discharge is normal. Expect a bright red flow of blood the first few days.

- If you've had an episiotomy or tear during vaginal delivery, there will be some soreness. Ask the nurse for an ice pack. Cold compresses and witch hazel pads reduce swelling. To take the sting out of urinating, squat rather than sit, and use a peri-bottle (most hospitals supply you with one). A peri-bottle is a squirt bottle. Fill it with warm water to squirt over your perineum while you are peeing. Refill the bottle and use it to cleanse your wound and vagina after each bathroom use. This promotes faster healing.

- Nurses will regularly monitor your baby, breastfeeding, vital signs, diaper changes, umbilical care, and teach you and your husband how to swaddle.

- The lactation specialist will visit, giving you and baby instructions and hands-on practice in breastfeeding, as well as answering any questions you may have. Over 50% of birthing women have epidurals, even if they deliver vaginally. Another side effect of the epidural is that your baby may have difficulty latching onto your breast. This was true with Alessio, and it took a good number of tries for us both to get proper feeding rolling.

All I wanted was to sleep, coddle and stare at the baby, and sleep some more. I was so glad that this was about all I had to do, thanks to those amazing nurses and dear Adriano, who stayed by my side on a little cot, and swaddled his son singing lullabies. Almost as important to my recovery, he brought me delicious meals from the restaurant across the street.

Pets and Newborns

If you have a dog at home and this is your first child, your pet will need some reassurance, since he is thoroughly convinced that *he* is your baby. I gave my sister one of Alessio's worn t-shirts to take home to my dog Bear, so he'd be familiar with the baby's smell and wouldn't be jealous or territorial. It worked like a charm.

If you have cats, it's best to begin baby training a few weeks before delivery. Teach your cat to stay out of the baby bassinette, stroller, and crib. How? Shoo him away whenever you catch your curious cat exploring baby territory. It's a myth that cats suffocate babies, but scratches are common—since a cat will playfully follow the baby's hand movements. Some cats like to chew on wool, and may be attracted to baby blankets.

Once you and your baby are home, be sure to keep your cat off counters where baby items are kept. Cats have bacteria in their mouths, as well as on their feet from cat litter. Prepare cat food in a separate place from baby food and bottle prep area. Disinfect counter tops regularly. Obviously, keep cat litter far from your newborn. Most cats are curious at first, then lose interest as the baby becomes part of the household.

Newborn Essentials

Borrow as many baby items as possible from friends.
Buy enough of the essentials to go a full week laundry-free.
Expect 2-3 outfit changes a day. My favorite kiddie stores:
Baby Gap, Diapers.com & The Children's Place.

☐ Onesies
- Wide/flexible neckline
- Breathable natural fabrics: cotton/bamboo
- Long & short sleeves

☐ Tops & Bottoms
- Wide/flexible neckline
- Long & short sleeves
- Elastic waistbands & full leg coverage

☐ Coats & Sweaters
- Soft & pliable enough for baby to move around
- Wide/flexible neckline
- Lightweight & heavyweight

☐ Socks & Shoes
- No-slip soles for socks
- Beginning to walk: shoes with flexible soles (to simulate being barefoot)
- Advanced walker: shoes with thicker sole & arch support

☐ Hats
- Lightweight hats for sleeping (first 3 months)
- Knit & sunshade hats for winter/summer walks

☐ Blankets
- Lightweight & heavyweight

☐ Diapers & Changing $
- Daytime & night diapers. Save money: buy in bulk.
- Wetness indicator tells you when baby needs changing.
- Diaper rash cream
- Wet Wipes (hypo-allergenic, fragrance- & alcohol-free)

☐ Grooming
- Baby nail clippers & file
- Baby toothbrush
- Baby hairbrush

☐ Lotion & Soap
- Fragrance-free
- Dermatologist approved for babies

☐ Infant Bathtub
- Digital water thermometer
- Tubs that fit in single or double sinks make bathing easier.
- Best design lets dirty water out while fresh water flows in.

☐ Hand Sanitizer
- For the first 2 months, family & friends should wash their hands before touching the baby.

$ = Money Saver

Chapter 13

Your New Normal

The first days home from the hospital with our firstborn Alessio, my husband and I were on what seemed an eternal treadmill of tasks: nursing every 2-3 hours day and night, changing diapers, swaddling, cuddling, soothing, burping, and more swaddling, interspersed with our complete exhaustion.

We were both feeling a little clueless, secretly thinking to ourselves: how could the doctor release dear Alessio from the hospital into our uncertain care? Just getting our newborn into the complicated car-safety seat without breaking his wobbly neck seemed a miracle.

We were full of questions. Alessio's belly button—was it healing properly? What about pacifiers? How would I know if he was eating enough, and was the crib really safe? How can we prevent SIDS, since nobody even knows what causes it? (Keep everything out of the crib—including blankets, and NEVER let your newborn sleep on her tummy, and even then parents worry....) I woke sometimes just to watch him sleeping and sometimes to check if he was breathing, then sometimes in a guilty rush if his tiny cries didn't wake me on the dot to feed him, dozing sometimes as I nursed him—then waking with a start, relieved to see that I hadn't smothered him with my gigantic breasts that were so painful I could barely touch them. Nursing was at times excruciating—not the cozy tender moments I had imagined when I was pregnant, which somehow felt a lifetime ago, though my belly still looked like I had yet to give birth.

Was our baby's penis healing correctly from the circumcision? What about his overbite, his lack of chin? My mother-in-law, Susan, was already imagining a chin implant for Alessio when he turned twelve. "Relax," my pediatrician said. "His chin will grow in. It's natural. All babies have it. The recessed chin allows better suction on the nipple." I began to realize Nature's genius and that even what we see as imperfections are perfect, despite my mother-in-law's fondness for improving on nature.

> Nature is a genius. What we see as imperfections are perfect in their own way.

I had the good fortune to have my mom, Adriano's mom, and my sister visiting the first week home from the hospital. Then my aunt and uncle showed up with enough food to feed an army (including one of my favorite's—Aunt Cathy's cheesecake). My dad and grandmother, Mama Lane, came too. So there were plenty of hands to hold the baby, change diapers, run errands, walk the dog and do dishes. And lots of discussions, too, about how to raise the baby, what was normal and what was not.

I couldn't believe that among my family, with a collective nine children between us, everybody had a different take. Even on burping! My mom did it one way, I was trained another, and Mama Lane said, "Lord! Don't you girls know anything about gas?!"

Maybe one reason we all had such different experiences and advice is that babies respond differently. Each one is unique, with his or her own particular temperament. Some are quiet. Some active. Some burp best on their tummies. Others like it over your shoulder. No method is right or wrong. It's a matter of preference—your baby's. What is your new normal? Your baby is your new normal, but what that entails you have yet to find out. One thing is sure: he'll be driving the household for the next few months. Get to know your baby's signals. They are talking all the time—from the moment they are born.

What Do Babies Know?

- At two days old, your newborn will begin to mimic your facial movements. Stick your tongue slowly in and out. See if your baby will follow your lead.

- Babies are active communicators. They show interest by slowed sucking or turning their heads toward whatever interests them. Even babies need time to be alone, and will tell you so—by turning away.

- Babies like baby talk. It seems they understand that the high-pitched sing-song sound is just for them, and prefer it over adult talk. Studies show that baby talk and the heightened emotions that go with it (did you ever see your face when you're talking to your baby?) help your child learn to communicate and understand language better.

- Be aware of how you speak in front of your baby. They understand what you are saying long before they can talk.

Source: Einstein Never Used Flash Cards

Managing the First Few Weeks

The first few weeks are crucial, both in your recovery from birthing, and adjusting to the baby and its needs. Your house is going to be a mess. Fine. So long as you are not. Friends will want to come over. Be protective of your time and energy. Make sure you schedule the visits with enough time for yourself. If friends ask what they can bring, tell them dinner or lunch. If they ask what they can do, dishes might be an option. Don't get caught playing the polite hostess when what you really need is a nap.

Give yourself three to six weeks to recover from birthing, especially if you've had a C-section. Pamper yourself as best you can during this hectic and wondrous time. Though it seems impossible, make time for you and your husband to bond, too, in your new roles. Steal time while baby is sleeping just to cuddle, and congratulate yourselves on how amazing you are as new parents. Most parents feel they are major screw-ups when even little things go wrong. Take it in stride. You are doing the best you can with what you know, and your learning curve is enormous. Remember: not only is your baby growing at the fastest rate of his lifetime—you and your partner are too.

Newborn Basics

- The average newborn sleeps 15-18 hours a day, and cries between 1-4 hours a day.

- For the first few weeks, babies need to nurse at least 8-12 times in a 24-hour period (about every 2-3 hours).

- Babies don't know if it's day or night. Neither do you at this point. Their tiny tummies don't hold much food, which is why they have to eat so often.

- You can't spoil a newborn. If your baby is crying, pick her up and see what she needs—even if it's just a cuddle.

My new-parent anxieties lessened when Alessio at two weeks old had his first visit with my pediatrician, Dr. Raker. As we were talking, she held him upside down and said, "Babies are very resilient. They really aren't that fragile." What a wonderful sense of relief I felt, watching my baby swimming on air!

Unexpected Joys

The motherhood guides I had read only politely hinted at the complete dysfunction between new parents—the lack of sleep mixed with anxieties and 24/7 responsibilities that create the nightmare cocktail of muddled conversations, loss of intimacy/identity, foggy thinking that in turn creates further anxieties and miscommunication, then deliberate withdrawal, the long silent moments staring into space, into the baby's face, into nothing you can remember anymore.

Any new parent will agree there are moments like this. Luckily they pass quickly into the fog. The first two months, I was stretched beyond limits I didn't even know I had, stretched farther than my belly had been. Two months into life, and my baby was still stretching me—farther into this new role of motherhood, far more demanding and rewarding than anything I had ever imagined.

My mom asked me if motherhood was what I had expected. I answered, "No. I didn't know I would laugh so much. I'm happier than I ever thought I could be—the baby gives me such joy." This I said after being up all night, Alessio in my arms and baby spit-up on my shoulder.

Teamwork: Organizing the Chaos. Your "new normal" is taking shape—both beautiful and challenging. Make this momentous transition as enjoyable as possible for everyone, including yourself. Don't put your needs on the back burner. A happy mom means a happy household. Sure, things will be bumpy at first. Try to find solutions to whatever might be bothering you, your baby or your husband. If something isn't working, change it.

Keep in mind that your mind isn't working as well as normal. We are a nation of sleep-deprived workaholics; new moms take that to an entirely new level. You will be forgetful and cranky and blissful. Sometimes all at the same time. Post-partum hormones also contribute to the haze, the craze, the bliss and sudden tears. It may seem weird to mention this, but take care of the little things—like brushing your teeth, showering, getting dressed. Find small ways throughout the day to refresh yourself—you're going to have to steal time, make more of it, spend what little you have in the best way possible.

Just because you're a new mom doesn't mean your personality has changed (though you may sometimes feel like Sybil). Try to organize your tasks according to your preferences. I hate shopping, so where I wanted help was the shopping for the week. I didn't mind meal prep; I was on for that task. I didn't mind light daily cleaning, but couldn't see where I had time or energy to actually do a weekly showdown with dirt.

If you can afford it, get help with your household tasks—even if only a few hours a week. If you can't, get comfortable letting things slide. No matter how clean your house habits used to be, a mess is better than exhaustion. Focus on you and the baby. Things will get done—eventually. And what doesn't, probably wasn't that important anyway.

Quick & Easy: Timesaving Shopping Tips

1. Keep an ongoing shopping list and favorite menus handy in the kitchen or on your computer, and modify them as needed. I try to add a new menu item each week to keep things fresh. If we like the new dish, it becomes a staple on our rotating menu of favorites. Use your menu list of ingredients to create your shopping list, so that dinners, shopping and meal prep for the week are planned out in one shot.

2. Try ordering groceries online and/or grocery delivery. A fully stocked fridge and pantry will give you peace of mind. Online shopping allows you to comparison shop to get the best deals. It also saves huge amounts of time.

3. You can buy all of your basic baby items online at Diapers.com. Convenient next-day delivery, with free shipping and no tax for most orders. Diapers, baby food, pacifiers—pretty much anything you need is available.

4. Buy enough baby bottles (around 8) and other daily-use essentials, so that you can go an entire day without having to wash anything.

5. For baby supplies used on a regular basis (diapers, formula, baby food), buying in bulk will save you money, time and energy. It might even give you enough time to treat yourself to a pedicure, now that you can see your feet.

Let Dad Do What He's Good At

Dads have a different way of relating to the baby, and are at a loss compared to the immense bonding Mom and newborn have had: nine months together in the same body. Is it any wonder he might feel a little left out? A common fear of new fathers is that you will love the baby more than you love him. A fear of being replaced. It can certainly seem that way as he watches you deliver, bond, nurse; the way the baby recognizes your voice first. Dads need their role in all of this, and to find what they are good at in the new balance of family life.

Adriano is an expert swaddler. He's proud of this and should be (I could never do it as well as he). Even the nurses at the hospital exclaimed that he was one of the best swaddlers they had ever trained. Was this true? Who knows? But learning to talk like that to your husband, as he fumbles and attempts to be a good dad—whatever that is (you both feel pretty clueless those first few weeks), is a good start. So praise him and hand the baby over. Let Dad do what he feels good about.

Lazy Husband Syndrome

What if your husband doesn't help as much as you need him to? Though things are changing for the better, it is still a common issue that most women routinely do more than their husbands at home, whether they work outside the house or not. It's called Lazy Husband Syndrome, but it is more complicated than that. Most men want to contribute, but at times they just don't know how. Believe it or not, men secretly think women do everything better. This often leads to an unspoken lack of confidence, especially around the house. As for women, we find it hard to ask for what we want, and often wait until we are angry before we ask for help. The combination can result in what many call the Chore Wars. Nagging doesn't work, though you might momentarily feel better. What does work?

Communication, negotiation, and cooperation. Ask for help and be specific. Show your appreciation. Never underestimate the power of a good word at the right time.

Moonlight Sonata—The Beauty of Routine

Prioritization, organization, and routines are key elements for creating a peaceful home. Setting routines for your family helps everyone adjust more gracefully to the pressures of new parenthood. Over time, your new routine will become second nature.

The first month, Adriano and I were both home. We divvied up baby-care in 3-hour shifts. Since we were both so exhausted, the short shifts were a great relief. We each knew when we were going to get a break to do whatever we wanted—nap, sit in silence, go for a walk. Down-time is important to gather your strength—don't fill it up with more to-do lists.

Work with your natural tendencies. Adriano was a night owl and I was a morning person. Once the baby had regained his birth weight, and I was producing enough breast milk, I took the night off sometimes. Before going to bed, I pumped enough breast milk so that Adriano could do the 3 a.m. feeding and I could sleep. Six a.m., I was up for the morning shift, while Adriano slept in.

If you are choosing to breastfeed, as long as you are producing enough milk, this arrangement works well. Keep in mind, pumping to skip a feeding can actually reduce milk production, since breastfeeding works on supply and demand. But exhaustion also reduces breast milk. It's a toss-up, but one thing is sure: a sleepless mom can be as dysfunctional as a texting driver wearing headphones. If you need a sleep break, take it.

Make family time part of your schedule. Adriano and I were both on duty from 4 in the afternoon until baby bedtime at 7 p.m. We went for family strolls, shared bath-time duties and read bedtime stories together. In the early evenings, Adriano and I listened to music like we'd always done—in the living room watching the fire, dancing sometimes. Now the three of us danced. Instead of putting ourselves aside for the baby, we enlarged our circle. It was a strange and wonderful thing, unexpected—the idea of expansion more than control. Enlarging our lives. We had to become more reliable for one another, more dependable, and trust each other to know what to do, even when we didn't actually know what to do. It was all navigating in the dark. A new road. New world.

Schedule time as a couple. While I nursed Alessio for his bedtime feeding, Adriano started dinner. Once the baby was down, I joined my husband in the kitchen, setting the table and mood for a candlelight dinner—where talking about baby was not on the menu.

Get your solo time. When you need to relax, hand the baby over to your partner and take a hot bath. Or take a walk around the neighborhood to clear your head.

Ask for help. Don't feel like a failure if things get to be too much. Whether you call a friend or a family member for back-up, do what you have to do to get through those first few tough weeks.

Let go of expectations. So the house is a mess, you haven't showered. It's okay. Learn to accept your "new normal." Remind yourself it won't be forever. Life will get back in order.

Baby Gear Essentials

I used the Orbit Infant Stroller System, which comes with a car seat that snaps into the stroller. Or use the Snap N Go Stroller, which allows almost any car seat to hook into the stroller. Read up on Car Seat Safety from the National Highway Traffic Safety Administration & Consumer Reports.

☐ Car Seat $

- High safety rating
- Can hook into your stroller, or use the Snap N Go Stroller
- Must be installed in car before baby comes home from hospital.

☐ Stroller

- Lightweight, compact, folds up & out easily
- Smooth suspension
- Good brakes, easy to set
- Adjustable handles
- Bag/place for storage
- Seat can recline all the way down for naps, & flip between rear-& forward-facing positions

☐ Baby Carrier

- Easy to put on & take off
- Can be worn as a front or back carrier
- Supports correct sitting position for the baby's hip, pelvis & spine growth

☐ Diaper Bag/Purse $

- Several pockets on the inside to separate your essentials from your baby's
- Save money: if you already have a large purse, just insert a purse organizer.

☐ Feeding & Sleeping $ Timer

- Portable with night light
- Multiple timers/settings so you can set reminders for feeding, changing & sleeping
- Save money: go digital by downloading a baby timer app.

$ = Money Saver

Chapter 14

When Do I Get My Body Back?

Good news! Your feet are shrinking. Bad news—your belly is not. At least not as fast as you had hoped. Nine months to put it on, and nine months to take it off, goes the saying. But that depends on your body and your lifestyle. If you stayed fit during pregnancy through healthy eating and daily exercise, it may take only six months to get back in shape. If you had a more sedentary lifestyle and not-so-great eating habits, it could take up to a year or more.

Happy Facts

- In childbirth alone, most women lose about 10 pounds—the sum weight of baby, fluids and placenta.

- Immediately after birthing, water retention becomes a thing of the past. As your body releases fluids over the next few weeks, you lose more weight, and get your ankles back, though your shoe size may remain about a half-size bigger than before.

- Your uterus, that had been 500x its normal size, only takes 6 weeks to get back to its pre-pregnancy size and muscle tone. (If only the rest of my body could behave that way!) Breastfeeding will speed the process along, as it causes the uterus to contract.

That's what is happening when you feel those strange twinges while you are nursing.

● Six weeks is the magic marker when you can have sex again. Whether you feel like it or not is another question. Breastfeeding lowers estrogen, so you may need lubrication. If you've had an episiotomy, your doctor will want you to wait until your postpartum checkup which is–take a guess!–at six weeks.

Getting into Shape

Deep breathing exercises can begin right away for all new mothers. It is a gentle way to reconnect with your body and begin strengthening your abdominal wall.

A few days after birthing, most women who have had a normal delivery can begin moderate exercise, such as walking and mild postpartum exercises. Begin slowly and work up to moderate walks three times a week. If you maintained daily exercise throughout your pregnancy, the general rule of waiting six weeks before strenuous exercise may not apply. Talk to your doctor. Listen to your body.

Stay Hydrated: If you are breastfeeding, keep in mind your fluid intake should increase to 13 cups (105 oz.) a day. Add an extra 1-2 cups for every half-hour of moderate exercise.

If you've had a C-section, about the only exercise recommended in the first six weeks after delivery are your Kegel exercises, which apparently every woman should do for the rest of her life.

● Don't lift anything heavier than your baby.

● Walking is great, as long as your body feels up to it.

● Get your doctor's approval before beginning any exercise program.

Abdominal Exercises: When your body is ready (6-8 weeks), start with gentle pelvic tilts, the bridge, and Kegels. Don't try to go from 0 to 100 in 60 seconds. Rebuild your strength with patience. Again, for moms who have had C-sections or stitches, get your doctor's approval.

Postpartum Surprises

Often women are so focused on having the baby, they miss being informed about the postpartum experience. Remember all the crazy things hormonal changes brought in the first trimester? In your first trimester of postpartum, hormones are shifting again, bringing some surprises that can be less than pleasant. Sweating is common, including night sweats for several months. Your body is eliminating fluids built up during pregnancy. Bleeding from the placenta area (whether you delivered vaginally or by C-section) lasts between 4-6 weeks and can be heavy at first.

Many women experience postpartum hair loss between three and six months after delivery. You won't go bald, but hair gets thin in places and may come out in clumps. Yes, you may hear the soundtrack for *The Good, the Bad and the Ugly* playing in your head, as a tumbleweed of hair rolls past you on your bathroom floor. Goodbye Beyoncé. Hello Baldi Locks. Rising estrogen levels gave you luxurious hair during pregnancy by making fewer hairs fall out. As hormones return to normal levels, the extra hair begins to shed. Women with long hair tend to notice this more. It's temporary and there are things you can do to smooth through it: keep taking your prenatals. Wash with a gentle conditioner. Use a gel or mousse that adds volume. Try a new hairstyle. Don't use dyes, bleaches, hair dryers or flat-irons.

Have patience. You will soon be through all of this before you know it, probably because you are too tired to notice the passing of time. But the baby in your arms speaks volumes that every moment you have gone through is worth it. (Except for the hair loss. Just kidding.)

When Do I Get My Mind Back?

Baby blues can strike even the cheeriest dispositions, affecting more than 50% of new mothers. It's a matter of those hormones again, along with the physical exhaustion of little sleep and birthing recovery. Again, the magic number is about 6-8 weeks for the blues to pass, and your strength and vigor to return.

If you're feeling blue, it's a good idea to make the time for some daily exercise. It works wonders in boosting mood and energy. Working out with fellow moms can also be a mood enhancer, plus get you motivated. Many health and community centers offer postpartum exercise classes.

Postpartum depression is different than baby blues, lasting longer with more severe mood swings. PPD affects about 10% of new moms, including those who were depressed before pregnancy. If you are feeling hopeless and the mood is severe and constant, contact your doctor and get the help you need. You will be glad you did.

Dieting, No Way! New Dress, Yes!

Forget diets. Your body needs the energy of good nutrition for recovery. Besides, weight lost too rapidly always returns. Don't discourage yourself by trying to squeeze into your old jeans before you are ready. But a few weeks postpartum is a good time to go shopping and treat yourself to a new dress or flattering new top in your new voluptuous mamma size. Make the most of your fabulous cleavage. Gap Body's line of elegant loungewear makes the perfect comfy daywear for postpartum recovery.

Chapter 15

Answers to Some of Those 1001 Questions

Diapers 101

For the first 2 weeks, use only water to clean baby during diaper changes. After 2 weeks, use alcohol-free baby wipes or soap and water. Wipes are great for cleaning up poo. For wet diapers, 4x4 gauze pads and water work just as well, and will save you money.

For girls, wipe front to back to prevent urinary tract infections. For uncircumcised boys, never push the foreskin beyond its natural limits. For circumcised boys: it takes about 1-2 weeks for circumcision to heal. Use Vaseline on the penis until healed, so it won't stick to the diaper.

If your baby has diaper rash, it's a sign you need to change her more often. Don't use baby powder—it's bad for a newborn's lungs. Use a diaper rash cream to speed up healing. Balmex is my favorite. Pampers Swaddlers Sensitive diapers have a wetness indicator line that makes it easy to know when your baby needs changing.

If your baby has a diaper rash, change his diaper more frequently.

Umbilical Care

It can take about 2-3 weeks for the umbilical cord to fall off. In the meantime:

- Give your baby only sponge baths (every other day is plenty).

- Keep the cord clean and dry. It's best left alone, but if it gets dirty, wash with soap and warm water. Gently dry with a clean cloth or fan with paper.

- Change diapers often, and make sure the cord isn't covered by the diaper.

- Call your doctor if cord is red, swollen, or oozing puss.

Baby's First Bath

Your baby's umbilical cord has finally fallen off and the navel is fully healed. It's time for another first—a bath.

- For the first time, it's a two-person job. The baby can be as slippery as a fish, and squiggly as one too. You'll likely need four hands. One person to firmly support the baby's head and neck, and keep him from sliding around, and the other person to wash, rinse and dry.

- Have everything you need handy: wash cloth, mild baby soap and shampoo, rinsing cup, soft cozy towel.

- Make sure the room is comfortably warm (75°F).

- BEFORE you put the baby in the tub, fill the tub with only 2-3 inches of water (from newborn to 6 months). Test the water temp. It should be about 85°F.

- Be prepared to get pee-d on if you have a boy. Keep that fire hose pointed downward as best you can. But if you do get an eyeful, it's comforting to remember urine is sterile.

- Go easy on the soap. Babies have sensitive skin. If your baby has eczema, which is common, use Cetaphil to wash.

- Most babies enjoy the water. Bathing can be a soothing bedtime ritual. I prefer bathing the baby in the early evening, followed by his feeding. He goes to sleep quicker and sleeps more soundly.

- If your baby isn't fond of water, choose an active time like morning to bathe.

- A counter-top baby tub that fits over the kitchen double sink worked best for me. The height made handling the baby much easier.

- Newborns only need bathed 2-3 times a week. Over-bathing will dry out their skin.

Safety Tips

- Never leave your child unattended—not even for an instant. Babies can drown in one inch of water. If you forget something or the doorbell rings, wrap your baby up and take her with you.

- Clear bathing area of electrical appliances.

- Set your water heater to less than 120°F. Scalding can happen in seconds.

Newborn Outings

For baby's first eight weeks, her/his immune system is still developing. While a walk around the block is good, definitely avoid crowded public areas such as the mall. When you go out, be sure the baby is comfortably dressed (not too hot or cold).

On one of my first outings with Alessio, like many new moms, I went overboard on the stroller prep—weighed down with diaper bag, burp rags, pacifier, toys, wet wipes, change of clothes. It looked like we were ready for a three-day expedition instead of a walk around the neighborhood. Alessio was so bundled up you could barely see his face. I had him securely wrapped in a plush straightjacket of sorts—his baby blanket combined with the seat belt that ran up through his legs and belted at his waist. Everything in place, including my sleep deprivation.

One thing I forgot to check: the stroller brake being fully engaged. As I turned to lock the door, I heard a click, click behind me. The stroller was rolling down the porch steps! I tried to grab the handles, but it was too late. The stroller flipped and fell. Alessio was inside, face-first on the sidewalk. I grabbed my baby and ran into the house crying, in a panic, sure that I had damaged my fragile little one for life. I handed the baby to Adriano to check if he was okay. I couldn't even look, I was so terrified. Amazingly, Alessio was fine.

In the forgetful first postpartum months, it helps to establish some good habits so you don't have to think too hard as you make your way through the day. A good habit on stroller operation: familiarize yourself with your stroller's latches, brakes, and seatbelt mechanisms—especially if the stroller basket can disengage from the carriage. Just like a car, a routine check before you get on the road is always a good idea.

Pacifiers and Thumb-Sucking

I was a constant thumb-sucker, so much that I had a callous on my thumb. Though my parents tried to break my habit, I didn't give it up until I was about three years old. My sister loved her pacifier so much they were inseparable. In almost every early photo of her, the pacifier was stuck to her face as if it were an appendage. Marisa basically only took it out to eat, then, plop, slurp slurp, back in it went. This went on until she was thirteen months old when, on a family picnic, she lost her revered friend. Another pacifier exactly the same would not do. She refused all but her beloved and rather crusty pacifier. After one night of crying it out, she said goodbye forever and never looked back.

Believe it or not, my mother sucked on a pacifier until she was seven years old. Her teeth are perfectly straight without braces. No palate problems either. Her mom never gave her grief about it (but her friends did). My grandmother, Mama Loma, was a free spirit who figured, "Hey, the kid probably knows more than I do." This being said, pacifiers were shaped differently than the ones used nowadays.

The sucking reflex is basic in babies. Many suck their thumbs or fingers, even in the womb. Pacifiers do the trick when your baby needs calming and are preferable to thumb-sucking (that's harder to wean). There is even some evidence that babies who sleep with pacifiers have a lower incidence of SIDS. Though some doctors warn that giving a pacifier will make your baby less interested in breastfeeding, it has not been my experience. Soothie First Year Pacifiers are recommended if you are breastfeeding. Latex-free, they are sized and shaped for a baby's developing mouth. They also cause the least amount of nipple confusion due to their naturally shaped nipple.

With my children, I try not to overuse the pacifier for calming, but when they need it, letting them suck and soothe is better than a crying fit. Nighttime and naptime, a pacifier gives the signal it's time to sleep.

Do pacifiers cause dental problems? According to Mayoclinic.com: "Normal pacifier use during the first few years of life doesn't cause long-term dental problems. However, prolonged pacifier use might cause a child's top front teeth to slant outward or not come in properly."

Most children naturally wean themselves from the habit, once they are ready. (Except my mom.) The average age for weaning is between two and four years old.

Chapter 16

Breastfeeding and Feeding Essentials

Breastfeeding

Breastfeeding is so beneficial for both baby and mother, all doctors recommend it for six months or longer, if possible. The antibodies and extreme nutrition of mother's milk improves your baby's brain and central nervous system development, and protects against a wide range of illnesses—including ear infections, respiratory illnesses, allergies, asthma, certain childhood cancers, urinary tract infections and major bacterial infections. Breastfeeding also decreases the incidence of diabetes, obesity and SIDS.

Health benefits for Mom include reduced risk of breast, ovarian and endometrial cancers, along with getting your body back into shape faster. Nursing speeds weight loss by burning calories. Oxytocin is released during breastfeeding, which makes the uterus contract and return to its pre-pregnancy size more quickly.

Not all moms feel the famous bonding rush.

Oxytocin, known as the "love and bonding hormone," is also released during sex and cuddling. The hormone is associated with monogamous behavior—

what scientists call "pair bonding," in addition to being credited for two other behaviors: "parental care" and "mate guarding." The genius of nature! If there was ever a time for bonding and commitment, it is the first few months of a baby's life when the child is completely dependent upon its parents for nurturing and survival. The bonding hormone plays a part in why you love to hold and stare at your baby. Oxytocin is released through skin-to-skin contact, and breastfeeding is about as skin-to-skin as you can get. Even if you are formula-feeding, skin time with your baby is important. Place baby on your breasts, tummy, bare arms. Skin is the body's largest organ, and emotional connection is transmitted through touch. Don't leave Dad out. Babies love to sleep on their dad's bare chest.

Not all moms feel the famous bonding rush. If you have concerns over bonding with your baby, be gentle. Give yourself time to adjust to all the changes. Try to spend more time with your baby—just sitting and playing, talking. Make time for skin-to-skin cuddling. If you have continued issues over bonding, you may have postpartum depression and should consult your doctor.

Another benefit of breastfeeding not to be ignored: it's free!

That said, most moms quit nursing at 3-4 months—when they go back to work. Our modern life doesn't quite mesh with the time and focus one needs for sustained nursing. Pumping at work is an option, but once the baby gets a taste of the easier sucking a bottle allows, he might prefer it to the breast—a phenomenon called "breast refusal."

Nonetheless, I made it my goal to breastfeed Alessio his first six months. I was determined to make it work, despite the challenges—including Alessio attacking my boob like it was a pint of Ben & Jerry's.

How It Works from Day One

New moms are encouraged to nurse as soon as possible after the baby is born, within the first hour if possible, which stimulates prolactin, oxytocin and milk flow. It will take several days for your milk to come in. In the meantime, from late pregnancy into birthing, you are producing colostrum, a low-fat high-carb protein filled with antibodies. Easily digestible, it is nature's perfect food for newborns, whose digestive systems are still developing in the first month or so after birth. Three to four days after birth, your mature milk will come in, and your breasts will gallop two cup sizes ahead overnight.

For the first few weeks, babies need to nurse at least 8-12 times in a twenty-four hour period (about every 2-3 hours). It's perfectly normal for a baby to take as little as five minutes or as much as an hour to complete a feeding, assuming that the baby is growing well (gaining 4-8 ounces per week in the first three months). Which is why your breasts will be sore for about the first week, proper latch or not. It's simply a lot of wear and tear on a very sensitive part of your body.

Try to nurse about 15 minutes per breast, or a minimum of 10 minutes. Keep the baby awake during feedings to help build stamina and routine.

The more your baby eats, the more milk you produce. It's a perfection of supply and demand. Release of prolactin, the hormone that regulates milk production in response to sucking, is greatest at night. That's why, no matter how insanely tired you are, do not skip night feedings until your milk flow is "established." What does that mean? Your milk production is steady, ample and your baby is showing all the signs of getting enough to eat: proper weight gain, diaper output, and increasing periods of alertness.

There is no way around it. For at least the first several weeks of your baby's life, you must surrender to the flow—the milk flow.

Quick & Easy: Ways to Boost Breast Milk

1 Drink lots of water.

2 Keep your diet nutrient-rich. Eat small, frequent meals. A nursing mom needs about 500 more calories a day than non-nursing women.

3 Get rest when possible. (Easier said than done with a new baby!)

4 Try mother's milk tea or fenugreek to boost your supply.

Newborn Weight Gain

Proper weight gain is crucial. Newborns lose weight the first 5-7 days. Five percent weight loss is normal for formula-fed; seven to ten percent weight loss is normal for breastfed. At 10-14 days, your baby should be back up to original birth weight.

Until your baby regains her birth weight, whether formula or breastfed, wake your newborn every 2-3 hours for scheduled feedings, 24/7. Feed on demand: if your newborn acts hungry before her next feeding is due, feed her. What are a baby's hunger cues? Sucking movements or sounds, rooting (turning head when cheek is stroked, and opening the mouth), wriggling or fussiness, rapid eye movement. What are a baby's *I'm friggin' hungry* cues? Tight fists, flexed arms, crying.

It's best to catch the early cues. If you wait until the baby is crying and tense, the baby is likely to suck harder on your already tender nipples. Also, if the baby is tense, proper latching is more difficult, along with digestion. There will be more gas and burping.

Newborns drink half their body weight in ounces per feeding. An 8 pound baby will consume 4 oz. of breast milk or formula.

What are the signs your baby has taken in all she wants at a feeding? Fists unclench, arms go limp, eyes haze over with a dazed, contented look—otherwise known as "milk drunk." How do you know that your baby isn't using your breast as a pacifier (appears to be milk drunk, but is still sucking)? Take the baby off your breast and burp her. If she starts to root again, it means she's still hungry.

During the first few months, babies will typically consume half of their body weight in ounces during a single feeding. For example, if your baby weighs 8 pounds, she will consume around 4 ounces of breast milk or formula.

Is Your Baby Getting Enough Milk?

The advantage to bottle feeding is that you know exactly how much formula your baby is taking in. For breastfed babies, tracking diaper output is one way to monitor if they're getting enough milk. Yes, new parents end up reading diapers as if they are tea leaves. By week one, a healthy newborn should be producing 4-6 wet diapers a day. Urine should be pale. If the urine is dark, it's a sign the baby needs more milk.

Over the first four days, infant poo will change from black to green to mustard color when mom's milk comes in. Consistency changes from sticky to loose. It doesn't stink much, but I'll warn you from experience, it can shoot across a room with the aim of a marksman and permanently stain white pants from 3 feet away. Breast milk is a laxative, so a nursing baby may produce as much as a stool each feeding. Formula-fed babies tend to poo less. At one month, your baby's digestive system is better developed and stools slow down. Normal can range from five times a day to once every five days.

Here's a quick reference chart to let you know if your baby is eating enough during the first week of life. There are a lot of free phone apps that you can download to track feedings and diaper output. My favorites are *Baby Activity Logger* and *Total Baby*.

Baby's Age	Urine Output	Bowel Movement	Color
Delivery Day	May have 1 wet diaper	May have 1 dirty diaper	Black, tarry, sticky
Day 1	1-2 wet diapers	At least one dirty diaper	Black, tarry, or dark green in color
Day 2	2 wet diapers	At least 1–2 dirty diapers	Dark brown–green in color
Day 3	2-3 wet diapers	1 or more dirty diapers	Green–brown in color, not as sticky
Day 4	4-6 wet diapers	1-10 dirty diapers	Brown–green–yellow in color and more runny
Day 5+	Soaking 6-8 diapers daily	3-10 dirty diapers daily	Mustard yellow, runny and seedy

The Proper Latch

The most important thing to know in breastfeeding is how to achieve a deep latch (baby's mouth properly positioned around your areola and nipple). Sounds simple, but not quite. The latching process depends on the shape of your breasts and nipple, and the baby's mouth size and sucking vigor, and how they fit together into a seamless happy milk flow. I'd been trained by a lactation specialist in the hospital, read a ton about breastfeeding, and had even taken a prenatal breastfeeding class at Cedars-Sinai, but after a week of breastfeeding, my nipples were cracked and sore (a sign the baby wasn't latching on properly and, therefore, likely not getting enough milk).

I made a date at the Pump Station, a local breastfeeding resource center, for an in-depth breastfeeding consultation with their specialist. She watched the baby nurse, then showed me a better way to hold him, and taught Alessio the right position to more deeply grasp the nipple. She also suggested a different nursing pillow. We then spent an hour doing practice-makes-perfect latching tries until Alessio and I both got it down.

Proper Latch Technique, straight from the Pump Station: "Baby should be latched about 1" below the nipple. It is usually better to be latched deeper under the nipple than above. The upper and lower lips should be flanged or curled out against the breast tissue. Baby's chin and cheeks should be slightly pressed to the breast, nose resting next to the breast." Latching tips: don't let the baby's head drop forward, or the lower jaw can't position deeply enough around the areola. It's easier to get into proper position if you're sitting up straight, using pillows.

The one-hour consult saved me weeks of pain. I went home with new confidence that just maybe I knew what I was doing, and breastfeeding soon became a pleasure.

Confidence is such a big factor in any kind of success. Breastfeeding is no different. Many new moms think breastfeeding, of all things, should come naturally, and are surprised at how awkwardly unnatural it feels at first. It's normal to have to work out a few kinks. Most communities have lactation specialists available. An excellent resource for nursing mothers is La Leche League at www.lalecheleague.org.

Breaking the Seal

How to remove baby from breast: insert your pinky into the corner of his mouth to break the seal. For vigorous suckers, you may need more than breaking the seal—get your finger right in there between the gums.

Tips for Sore Breasts

- Spread your breast milk over the nipple, before and after nursing. Works amazingly well!

- Motherlove ointment combined with Ameda ComfortGel Hydrogel Pads. This combination really reduced the irritation. Within a week my nipples were back to normal.

- Begin feedings on the least sore nipple.

- Breastfeed every 2-3 hours for short periods (5-7 minutes).

- Allow the nipples to air dry after each feeding.

- Wear softshells in your bra.

- If nipples are cracked, use a pump instead.

- Wear a nursing bra 24 hours a day.

How to Tell if Breastfeeding is Going Well

- Baby feeds at least 4-5 times in first 24 hours.

- Baby will sustain latch and suck for at least 5 minutes, preferably 10-15 minutes.

- Mother's nipples do not hurt nor are they misshapen after a feed.

- Baby has produced at least one stool and one wet diaper per 24 hours since birth.

If You Pump, Breast Milk Will Stay Good

- 4 hours at room temperature

- 4 days in fridge

- 4 months in freezer

If you are bottle feeding in the early months, use slow flow nipples, especially if you are using a bottle and breastfeeding. Reason: bottle flow is faster, and breast milk slower. The baby may prefer the easier suck. Also faster milk flow may be too much for your newborn's tiny tummy.

Nursing Comfort Station

You'll be surprised how fast you get the hang of it, once you learn, not only proper feeding techniques, but to trust your motherly instincts—which will grow naturally as you spend time with your baby. Make breastfeeding a wonderful experience by creating a welcoming space where you can relax and settle into it. Set up everything you'll need: a comfortable chair, back pillows and nursing pillow, footrest, table in reach with water, your phone, tissues, burp rags, a good book or music, a snack. The more relaxed you are, the easier your milk "lets down."

Nutrition and Breastfeeding

For good milk production, stay hydrated. Drink a full glass of water with each feeding. To increase milk production drink Mother's Milk tea. Keep taking your prenatal vitamins, and follow the basic healthy eating guidelines from Chapter 3.

You can have alcohol, but don't drink right before breastfeeding. A glass of wine takes 2-3 hours to metabolize. If you want some wine, have it right after you nurse. Moderate caffeine intake is okay for most breastfeeding moms and does not affect most babies.

Though you can eat pretty much anything, your baby may react to what you've had for supper. I love broccoli and brussel sprouts, but Alessio had a different take. He was up all night crying with gas.

If you are formula feeding, it's still a good idea to keep taking your prenatals and eat healthy, especially through the 6-8 weeks your body needs to recover from childbirth.

Quick & Easy: Breastfeeding Tools for Success

1. Breast shells, if you have flat or inverted nipples, will help the baby latch on correctly and protect your nipples if they are irritated.

2. Pillows. I tried a variety. My favorite was the Luna Lullaby. Another favorite for many of my friends is My Brest Friend pillow.

3. Itzabeen Timer or a Smartphone App that tracks when the next feeding is due, and how long baby feeds at each breast. It also has a switch to remind you which breast you fed from last.

4. Breast Pump: there are 2 types—manual and electric. The manuals are less expensive, and also take longer to pump smaller amounts. Electric works faster and costs more. A double pump allows you to pump both breasts at the same time, which is convenient, especially if you are pumping at work. Medical supply stores rent pumps for $1-3 a day. I borrowed a Medela double pump from my sister-in-law with my first baby. I liked it so much, with my second baby I bought my own.

Introducing Solid Foods

When your baby is 4-6 months old, you can give her water and start to introduce solid foods. It's best to start juices later, due to their high sugar content. Infants usually like cereals, fruits (like mashed bananas) and sweeter vegetables, like carrots and sweet potatoes. But don't neglect other vegetables. Introduce a variety of foods. The new pediatric recommendations are that a wider variety of foods can help prevent allergies. No more rules about at a certain age, certain foods should be introduced. Any and all foods are considered okay to give your baby, starting at about 6 months old (except raw honey). So yes, you could give your 6 or 8 or 10 month old peanut butter or yogurt. If your baby doesn't like a particular food, try reintroducing it later. It can take a few tries.

Raw honey is the only exception to the new food rules. Raw honey should not be given to your baby until a year old.

As solids are introduced, breast milk and formula consumption levels change. Your baby's liquid intake will decrease as solids increase. A good rule of thumb with solids is to alternate food groups with each feeding to ensure your baby is getting a balanced diet.

Start with solids once or twice a day, and finish each meal with nursing or a bottle. Some babies prefer a little formula first to take the edge off their hunger. Let your baby eat as much as she wants. Don't force a baby to eat.

As solid intake increases, most babies settle into a pattern of 3 meals of solids each day. The amount of formula tends to drop off, but typically stays in the range of 6-8 ounce bottles, 3 to 5 times a day. A smaller bottle (or half a bottle) is given with each meal, and a larger one at bedtime. Some babies also enjoy a bottle first thing in the morning.

An older baby (8-12 months) can have up to 32 ounces of formula per day, in addition to water, juice and solids.

My original goal was to feed Alessio only homemade food starting at 6 months. I bought the Beaba Babycook Baby food maker. I cut up fruits and vegetables, steamed, then mashed them. I did this for the first few weeks, but the Babycook was hard to use and I burned myself a couple of times. Then I discovered Earth's Best jarred food. When I read the ingredients and realized they were all organic, and that Alessio preferred the taste of the jarred food over my home cooking, I switched and gladly. According to my pediatrician, with the new eating rules, even purees are not absolutely necessary anymore for babies 6 months and older. My take is that gradual introduction of easily digestible foods is smart to start, then go from there.

From 6-8 months: When introducing solids, start slowly. Offer a tablespoon of cereal after your child has finished the breast milk or formula. Solids should not replace milk. Breast milk or formula is still the primary source of nutrition through the first year. Feed a single food for 3-4 days to see if your baby has any allergic reactions. Within 2-3 months of starting solid foods, your baby will be eating three solid meals per day. This is also a good time to introduce a sippy cup.

At 8-10 months: Finger foods are a favorite, as your baby will be grabbing things and learning hand-to-mouth coordination. Your baby's formula intake will decrease to about 20–24 oz. per day and breastfeeding may decrease to 4-5 times per day.

By 10–12 months: By 10-12 months, your baby may be weaning from breast milk or formula to whole milk. Help ease the change by offering ½ breast milk and ½ milk, or ½ milk and ½ formula blend during the first few days of the transition. Whole milk has a lot of fat that is good for brain development; 16-24 oz /day provides an adequate amount of calcium. Continue to wean the bottle and encourage a cup.

Feeding Chart for Baby's First Year

Feeding Chart: 0-4 Months

BREASTMILK	AMOUNT: At least 10-12 times within a 24-hour period. Every 2–2 ½ hours for the first couple of months. A baby should consume up to half his weight in ounces in a single feeding. If your baby weighs 8 pounds, offer him 4 ounces.
FORMULA	AMOUNT: At least 10-12 times within a 24-hour period. Every 2½ to 3 hours. INTAKE RANGE: 18–40 oz per day **Quick Tips** • When mixing formula, add the water first, then add formula and shake. • If you are feeding with a bottle, feed in the upright position. • Most newborns want to eat every 2-3 hours. Start with 1-2 oz at each feeding the first week, then work up to 2-4 oz. As your baby gets older and his tummy gets bigger, he'll drink fewer bottles a day with more formula in each. In a couple of months, he may be down to 6-8 bottles of 4-6 oz every 24 hours, depending upon your baby's intake range. • A baby should consume up to half his weight in ounces in a single feeding. If your baby weighs 8 pounds, offer him 4 ounces.
SOLIDS—None	No cereals, grains, fruits, vegetables, protein or dairy.

Feeding Chart: 4-6 Months

BREASTMILK	AMOUNT: At least 10-12 times within a 24-hour period. Every 2½ to 3 hours.
FORMULA	AMOUNT: At least 10-12 times within a 24-hour period. Every 2½ to 3 hours. INTAKE RANGE: 24-45 oz per day **Quick Tips** • Offer your baby 2.5 oz of formula per pound of body weight. • By 4 months, she'll probably drop to 4 or 5 bottles of 6-7 oz each. By 6 months, she'll typically be down to 3 or 4 bottles of 7-8 oz each a day.
SOLIDS	AMOUNT: .16 oz or 1 teaspoon of cereal or other easy to digest solid with .66-.83 oz. or 4-5 teaspoons of breast milk or formula twice a day.

Feeding Chart: 6-8 Months

BREASTMILK	AMOUNT: As frequently as baby demands (at least every 3–4 hours), along with solids
FORMULA	AMOUNT: Up to 37 oz per day, with solids INTAKE RANGE: 24–37 oz per day **Quick Tips** Give your baby a bit of formula before feeding her the solid food, to take the edge off her hunger. Once she finishes the solids, try giving her a bit more formula to see if she is still hungry. Give a full bottle (8 oz) before putting her to bed.
SOLIDS Cereals & Grains	AMOUNT: .5-2.5 oz or 1–5 tablespoons mixed with formula per day **Quick Tips** When starting baby on cereals, feed one type of grain at a time to make sure there are no allergic reactions. If your baby takes them well, you can try mixing them together for variety of taste and nutrients. OPTIONS: Rice, barley, oats
Fruits	AMOUNT: 2-4 oz or 4–8 tablespoons per day **Quick Tips** Begin making your own fruit combinations once baby has had several fruits without any allergic reaction(s). OPTIONS: Avocado, apples, bananas, apricots, mangos, nectarines, peaches, pears, plums, prunes, pumpkin

Feeding Chart: 6-8 Months, con't.

Vegetables	AMOUNT: 2-4 oz or 4–8 tablespoons per day **Quick Tips** Time for some veggie combos. Make sure your baby has tried all the vegetables first, and had no reactions, prior to mixing & matching. If your baby doesn't like something at first, give it a few tries. Babies' tastes change as they mature. OPTIONS: Sweet potatoes, acorn/butternut squash, carrots, green beans, peas, yellow squash/zucchini, parsnips
Protein	AMOUNT: 1-2 oz or 2–4 tablespoons per day **Quick Tips** Try offering tofu finger cubes dusted with cereal "dust" (helps baby grasp slippery foods). Many pediatricians now recommend meats as first foods, due to the iron content. OPTIONS: Turkey, chicken, tofu
Dairy	AMOUNT: 1–2 oz or 2–4 tablespoons per day **Quick Tips** Babies love yogurt and mild cheeses. Mix yogurt with a favorite fruit puree for a breakfast treat.

Feeding Chart: 8-10 Months

BREASTMILK	AMOUNT: As frequently as baby demands (at least every 4-5 hours), along with solids
FORMULA	AMOUNT: Up to 31 oz per day with solids INTAKE RANGE: 24–31 oz per day
SOLIDS Cereals & Grains	AMOUNT: 1.5–2.5 oz or 3–5 tablespoons mixed with formula per day **Quick Tips** • Begin offering breads and muffins when baby has mastered mashed and more textured foods. • Pasta makes a great finger food. OPTIONS: Flax, graham crackers, kamut, quinoa, millet, multi-grain, crackers, whole grain Cheerios, wheat & wheat germ, toast
Fruits	AMOUNT: 2-4 oz or 4–8 tablespoons per day **Quick Tips** • Try offering raw, ripe fruits. • Soft-cooked fruits make great finger foods. OPTIONS: Blueberries, cantaloupe & melons, cherries, cranberries, dates, figs, grapes (peeled and mashed into other foods only), kiwi, papaya

Feeding Chart: 8-10 Months, con't.

Vegetables	AMOUNT: 2-4 oz or 4–8 tablespoons per day **Quick Tips** • Soft-cooked veggies make great finger foods. • Try mixing up a veggie medley. Add grated cheese for extra yum. • Sauté or roast onions or peppers to add to baby's food, or serve as finger foods. OPTIONS: Asparagus, broccoli, cauliflower, eggplant, white potatoes, onions, peppers, leeks, mushrooms, parsnips
Protein	AMOUNT: 1-2 oz or 2–4 tablespoons per day **Quick Tips** • Continue to offer a variety of foods. An omelet is the perfect chance to slip in some veggies. OPTIONS: Eggs, beans/legumes, beef, chicken, pork, ham, fish
Dairy	AMOUNT: 2-3 oz or 4–6 tablespoons per day **Quick Tips** • Get adventurous with cheeses and yogurts. Avocado mashed with a bit of cream cheese. Mmm! OPTIONS: Cream cheese, cottage cheese, colby jack, cheddars

Feeding Chart: 10-12 Months

BREASTMILK	AMOUNT: As frequently as baby demands (at least every 4-5 hours), along with solids
FORMULA	AMOUNT: Up to 31 oz per day with solids INTAKE RANGE: 24–31 oz per day
SOLIDS Cereals & Grains	AMOUNT: 2.5–4 oz or 5-8 tablespoons mixed with formula per day **Quick Tips** Break out the shaped pasta. Create your own baby pasta salad with favorite veggies and cheeses. OPTIONS: Pastas, wheat cereals, bagels
Fruits	AMOUNT: 2-4 oz or 4–8 tablespoons per day **Quick Tips** Go slowly if introducing citrus fruits. Watch for possible reactions to acidity. OPTIONS: Berries, cherries, citrus, dates, grapes (cut in quarters to avoid choking hazard)
Vegetables	AMOUNT: 2-4 oz or 4–8 tablespoons per day **Quick Tips** Try mixing up a soft-cooked, diced veggie medley. Slowly introduce tomato and other acidic foods. Watch for reactions to the acidity. OPTIONS: Artichokes, beets, corn, cucumbers, spinach, tomatoes

Feeding Chart: 10-12 Months, con't.

Protein	AMOUNT: 1-2 oz or 2–4 tablespoons per day **Quick Tips** My babies love baked fish plain or breaded. Offer with steamed veggies for a healthy meal.
Dairy	AMOUNT FOR 10-12 MONTHS OLD: 3 oz or 6 tablespoons per day AMOUNT FOR 12 MONTHS OR OLDER: 16–24 oz per day OPTIONS: Whole milk as a drink, stronger cheddars, gouda, munster, provolone, swiss, feta, brie
Sweeteners	When baby is 12 months, you can introduce raw honey

Sources: American Academy of Pediatrics, Pump Station, Sanford Health, Wholesome Babyfood.com

Feeding Essentials

☐ Nursing Bra
- Gives support & prevents nipple irritation (bring to hospital)
- Comfortable with no underwire
- Clips at front, next to straps
- Lower cut so you can wear a variety of tops

☐ Breastfeeding Relief $
- Nipple cream (bring to hospital)
- Gel pads to wear under your nursing bra (bring to hospital)
- Hot & cold presses

☐ Breastfeeding Pillow
- Flexible support to fit any body type
- Pillow cover (removable & washable)

☐ Breast Pump $
- Adjustable suction levels & double-pumping capability
- Hands-free breast pump bra
- Breast milk storage bags

☐ Bottles
- BPA-free
- Designed to reduce air bubbles
- Easy to clean
- Slow-flow nipples for first 4 months (faster flow thereafter)

☐ Bottle Drying Rack
- Enough slats to dry 8 bottles & accessories

☐ Bottle Warmer
- Automatic shut-off

☐ Formula
- Main types of formula: cow's milk, soy milk & protein hydrolysate.
- Talk to your pediatrician about the right one for your baby.

☐ Solid Food
- Make your own solids in a blender or buy jarred baby food.
- Go for natural & organic.
- Variety of cereal, fruits (prunes for constipation), veggies & protein

☐ Burp Cloths & Bibs
- Lots! Expect to use 2-3 a day.

☐ Sippy Cups, Spoons, Forks & Bowls
- BPA-free
- Introduce solids & sippy cups when your baby is 6 months old.

☐ High Chair
- Adjustable tray & footrest
- Easy to clean

$ = Money Saver

Chapter 17

Fussy Baby

On average, a newborn cries between one to four hours a day. Frazzled parents will be happy to know that crying peaks around two months and steadily declines from thereon in. Why do babies cry? It's not just to further unravel what little you have left of your sanity. Crying is your baby's means of telling you something.

Believe it or not, sometimes babies cry just to release emotional stress. Yes, your little one really *is* a little person, and we have more in common than we think with our infants. Sometimes babies cry because they are lonely or bored and need more stimulation. Other times, they cry because they are over stimulated and want to be left alone.

Newborns cry 1-4 hours a day. Crying peaks at 2 months and declines from there.

How does a mother know what her baby is trying to tell her, when her child can only communicate with smiles, tears, gurgles, grunts, groans, fists flying, feet kicking and a few well-placed hiccups, burps and toots? Is it true there are different cries for different needs? Does pitch and volume indicate anything other than the healthy lung capacity of your newborn?

Over time you will begin to understand the varying cries and body language of your newborn. But initially, deciphering your baby's codes is a process of trial and error, which I prefer to call trial and solution. Spend time observing your newborn. In my first few weeks of new motherhood, I would just lie in bed with Alessio and talk to him, watch his reactions and try to understand his different mannerisms. This helped me better understand his cues.

When he was sleepy, he had a tendency to rub his eyes. Hunger produced a firmer, more insistent cry. If he needed to suck for soothing, he signaled me with his little tongue and the way he opened his lips. I tried to catch his messages before the tears began. Once a baby is upset, it can take some time to quiet down.

When your baby cries, remain calm and try to figure out what is bothering her. If you pick her up and she stops crying, it's likely she just wanted company or stimulation. Many babies like to be swaddled. Swaddling mimics the snug safety of the womb and calms some babies down. If holding or swaddling doesn't work, remember most babies cry for one (or more) of the following reasons:

- Hungry

- Tired

- Need a diaper change

- Gassy

- Acid reflux

- Too hot or cold (add or remove clothes)

- Need to suck for soothing (try pacifier or clean pinky)

In the early weeks, the more you cuddle and coo, the better. You can't spoil newborns. If they cry to be held, it's because they need to be held. You can trust your baby is telling the truth when you hear her little voice (sometimes not so little) calling you for assistance.

Signs Your Baby May Have Gas

Face it. Everyone on earth experiences gas, and newborns more so because their digestive systems are still developing. Breastfed babies usually have less gas than bottle-fed babies. If your baby has gas, don't look for the obvious toots and belches, which in baby terminology spells "relief." The signals to look for are:

- Crying for no understandable reason. Cries may be sharp and erratic.

- Discomfort: squirming, grimacing, kicking or pumping legs.

- Hiccups (caused by air pockets forming in the baby's stomach).

Quick & Easy: Ways to Reduce Gas

1   If you are breastfeeding, burp your baby when switching breasts.

2   If bottle-feeding, burp your baby every 2-3 minutes during feeding for the first few weeks. By one-month old, burp your baby when bottle is half-finished.

3   Hold your baby upright a few minutes after feeding, before you lay him down.

4   Don't overfeed your baby. Follow this formula: baby's weight$\div 2$ = maximum ounces per feeding. (An 8-pound baby should get 4 oz. max per feeding.)

5   Sugar causes more gas in babies. Avoid formulas with sugar.

6   Breastfed babies react to mom's diet. Spices, citrus, gassy veggies, and chocolate are common gas factors. Look for your baby's digestive patterns in what you eat.

7   Swallowing gets rid of hiccups. Try a quick feeding, some gripe water, or a pacifier.

Best Ways to Burp

There are a number of ways to burp your baby. All of them work, but often your baby will respond more favorably to a specific position. The most common is to hold your baby against your chest, with her chin above your shoulder, and gently pat or rub her back. The rubbing motion can be circular or up and down. You are trying to move gas out of the baby's system.

You can also sit your baby on your lap, and lean him slightly forward, supporting his chest and head with one hand. Gently pat or rub his back. If this position doesn't do the trick, try placing your baby on your lap, on his stomach, and pat or rub his back. Some babies respond to more vigorous patting, near the rump.

Another effective method is to lay your baby on her back, and move her legs in a circular motion, like riding a bike.

Medicinal Remedies

- **Wellements Gripe Water:** All natural with a 95% success rate in easing gas, colic and tummy ache. Available from health food stores, practitioners' offices and on-line. The only downside: it needs refrigeration.

- **Mylicon:** Made from simethicone, it isn't as natural as gripe water but is easier to use on the go, as it doesn't require refrigeration. Never give more than the recommended dose.

- **Baby's Jarro-Dophilus:** The vegetarian formula contains probiotics that help babies' digestion. For Alessio's first 3 months, I mixed it with gripe water. Jarro-Dophilus can also be added to formula. If you prefer, talk to your pediatrician about formulas with probiotics in them.

Infant Acid Reflux

Babies do their fair share of spitting up after eating. One reason is the muscle between the esophagus and stomach, which controls swallowing, is still developing. Infant acid reflux (GER) affects most babies to some degree. Symptoms include spitting up, coughing, wheezing, crankiness around feeding times, and crying—especially when lying on his or her back after a feeding. Infants normally grow out of the condition between 12 and 18 months old.

What you can do: feed your baby more frequently and smaller amounts. Burp during feedings. Try other feeding positions. Infant acid reflux happens to healthy babies and does not affect growth or wellness.

If your baby's symptoms are more severe and he/she is not gaining weight, is spitting up with force or vomiting, or refuses to eat, contact your doctor. These may be signs of the more serious condition, gastroesophageal reflux disease (GERD).

Colic

Colic affects up to 25% of babies. It is best described as an attack of crying and what doctors believe to be abdominal pain. Nobody actually knows what causes colic. According to Mayo Clinic, "Researchers have explored a number of possibilities, including allergies, lactose intolerance, an immature digestive system, maternal anxiety, and differences in the way a baby is fed or comforted."

One theory for relief is to maintain a peaceful household. This means avoid having anxiety, anger or fear in the house. Good advice for anyone.

The good news is that colic isn't harmful to your baby and has no long-term effects. A baby with colic will gain weight and eat normally. If your baby has repeated episodes of inconsolable crying for more than 3 hours in 24 hours, he may have colic.

Colic babies usually cry at the same time of day—often afternoon or evening. Symptoms include tight fists and tensed abdominal muscles. Keep in mind that some babies have regular crying hours, and some babies need to cry a little to get to sleep—this does not mean your child has colic. Pay attention to your child's patterns to understand if it's colic or something else. When in doubt, contact your pediatrician.

Colic generally begins several weeks after birth and is over between 3-4 months of age. If you are the parent of a baby with colic, get a calendar and start counting down the days. Remind yourself: life is ever changing. You will make it through. One day (far in the future) you may even laugh.

I have a friend who had colicky twin boys. Jennifer said there was a time when she thought she was losing her mind. One day she was driving with her boys, who were crying uncontrollably. She pulled over and stepped out of her car, took a lot of deep breaths and cried. Colic is a phase not a life-sentence, she reminded herself. It would be over in a couple of months. She held onto that thought as she got back in her car.

Moms need to know when to take a break. If you feel you are at your limits, do the same as my friend: make sure your child is safe, then step back and breathe deeply until your calm returns. If you need help, call a friend or your doctor. Remember, this too shall pass. It's not only your baby who sometimes needs a good cry.

The Hunger Quotient

At 5:30 p.m. every day, my newborn wailed a storm. The rest of the day Sienna was all smiles, but at 5:30, as if she possessed a Swiss watch, the wailing began. I went down my checklist. She was fed, burped, diapers changed, not hot or cold, pacifier in place. I tried swaying, swinging, swaddling, strolling. She would have none of it. And the megaphone voice on that child!—insisting on something I just wasn't getting.

So I called my doctor, who simply said the first thing on my list: "Maybe she's hungry." But I had fed her, right on time, 3:30 as usual, I explained. (I have my own Swiss watch mentality about organization and routine, especially around feeding). Sienna had shown all the signs of being sated—milk drunk, limp hands, dazed eyes, contentment—not to mention she had proper weight gain. All the *should's* checked right down the line.

My doctor said, "There's only one way to find out. Give her an extra ounce of stored breastmilk or formula after her feeding. If she drinks it, you'll know that she is not getting enough at the breast and needs a little more at each feeding." My baby downed the full ounce. With that brilliant insight, Sienna's wailing days were over.

Constipation

When Alessio was six-months old, we introduced solid foods. Constipation instantly set in. We gave him extra water and fruit juice to no avail. Two days and counting, my pediatrician told me to gently swab his bum with the tip of a cotton swab dipped in Vaseline. Nada. Next step: a pediatric glycerin suppository. Bingo! From no-go to whoa-whoa. The suppository worked within fifteen minutes. A little too well. I swear I couldn't figure how such a small tyke could manufacture enough poop to smear half-way up his back, through his diapers, and right onto a white leather couch.

For the next two months, Alessio got prunes every morning to regulate his system.

Plum Organics prunes are perfect for everyday and travel. They come in an easy-to-transport pouch. I also used Earth's Best prunes, and tried my own hand at puréeing prunes with a lot of water. Bottom line: any prunes will do as long as they are pit-free.

Feed babies (over 6 months old) high-fiber baby foods, if they are easily constipated. Avoid rice cereal, bananas, applesauce and starchy foods. Try barley cereal, prunes and plums.

The Poop Scoop: What is Normal?

If a baby's stool is hard and dry, it is considered constipation, even if the bowel movement is regular. If your newborn is constipated, call your doctor. If your baby is six months or older, give him extra water or fruit juice—this does not replace breast milk or formula feeding.

Constipation is normal when a baby switches from breast milk to formula, or from milk to solid foods. Do not use laxatives, mineral oil or enemas.

If your older baby is constipated, try a change in diet first. Infant glycerin suppositories are for occasional use, when dietary changes do not work. As always, if the condition persists, contact your pediatrician for advice.

Teething

Last but not least, another common Fussy Baby factor is teething. First teeth usually sprout between 3-12 months; typically the bottom middle teeth. The average age to begin teething is six months. By two years old, your child's last teeth will begin to appear (top and bottom back molars). By three years old, most children's full set of twenty baby teeth are complete.

These are averages. Every child is different. Some babies are born with teeth. Others take a full year to show off their new choppers.

Want to know if your baby is teething? Slide your clean pinky along her gums. If you feel a small bud below the surface, then yes. Also, look for "whitecaps"—the sharp ridge of a new tooth breaking through. Often though, before anything shows up, your baby will let you know in other ways. Signs to watch for:

- Lack of appetite

- Drooling

- Fever

- Gnawing

- Tender gums

My favorite remedy is Boiron Camilia Teething Relief, an all-natural homeopathic solution that contains rhubarb (for digestion), chamomile (for pain) and pokeweed (for gums). Even with homeopathic medicines, do not exceed the recommended dose. Boiron Camilia is affordable and available in stores and online.

Teething toys work wonders! Be sure to have a variety on hand. They come in soft, medium and hard, as your baby will have differing needs according to the teething stage. Some can be refrigerated so they have a cooling effect on your baby's gums.

Comfort Zone

Infant Massage

Massage is common practice for preemies, but full-term babies can benefit too. It helps them sleep better and grow faster. Try a gentle foot rub, or laying your baby on his back and raising his arms above his head, then down. Cycle the legs like riding a bicycle.

Swaddling and Shushing

Most babies like to be swaddled (at about four months old they outgrow the need). Swaddling recreates the familiar safety of the womb, and can instantly soothe a fussy baby. Shushing (a rhythmic whisper similar to "hush") can also calm your infant. According to Dr. Harvey Karp (*The Happiest Baby on the Block*), shushing imitates the whoosh of blood pumping through the womb, a comforting sound your baby knows.

Top Five Baby Pleasers

- Play with your baby: dance, sing, talk, read.

- Babies like movement. Try gentle rocking and swaying, or an infant swing.

- Babies like to gaze at brightly colored objects, and black-and-white contrasting patterns. Try a mobile or place baby where he can see the play of sunlight and shade on a wall.

- Babies like variety. For stimulation, park baby's bassinette near household activity. For quiet time, near the gentle flow of a fountain or other white noise.

- Babies like music. Even newborns have their favorites. Play a few tunes and discover which ones your baby likes by watching her reaction.

Quick Tip Checklist For Your Fussy Baby

Hungry	If your newborn hasn't eaten in 2 hours, she may be hungry—even if it's not her regular feeding time.
Tired	Newborns sleep between 15 and 18 hours a day. If your baby hasn't slept in the last hour, she probably needs a rest.
Dirty Diaper	Newborns produce about 10 wet diapers a day, and up to 10 poo diapers. Luckily it tapers off after several weeks. Check your baby often.
Gassy	Burp by patting or rubbing the back. For hiccups, get baby to swallow: give gripe water or a quick feeding.
Acid Reflux	Feed your baby more frequently and smaller amounts. Burp during feedings. Try other feeding positions.
Temperature	Check baby's hands to see if they are hot or cold. Adjust clothing accordingly.
Stimulation	Your baby may fuss because he needs company or variety: pick him up, coo and cuddle, or take him for a walk in the stroller. Likewise, your baby may fuss because he is over-stimulated: move him to a quiet, calm place.
Soothing	Babies have a need to suck for soothing. Try a pacifier or clean pinky. Babies also respond to swaddling, shushing and white noise.
Teething	Is your baby drooling a river, coupled with a loss of appetite? Don't worry. The likely culprit is a new tooth. Teething can begin as early as 3 months. Baby will be cranky from the pain, and may also have sleep disruptions. Use extra love, teething toys, gentle gum massage, and natural pain relief. Teething bouts usually last a few days.

Fussy Baby Essentials

☐ Gas Relief

- During the first 4 months, your baby will experience gas.
- Make sure you have plenty of gas relief on hand.
- Gripe water works wonders!

☐ Teething & Pacifier

- Natural teething relief, such as Boiron Camilia
- Pacifier & teething toys help relieve teething pain.

☐ Anti-Allergy Medicine

- Best not to use before 6 months of age.
- Keep on hand in case your baby is allergic to any new solids introduced to his/her diet.

☐ Cough & Cold

- Nasal aspirator/suction
- Saline drops/spray
- Fever reducer. For babies under 6 months use acetaminophen; for babies over 6 months, use either ibuprofen or acetaminophen.
- Traditional oral or temple thermometer. (Ear thermometers don't work on newborns.)
- Warm-air humidifier with different moisture release settings & auto off-function

☐ The Happiest Baby on the Block DVD $
by Harvey Karp, M.D.

- Provides tips on calming crying babies & how to swaddle & soothe.
- Save money: rent the DVD or check it out from your local library.

$ = Money Saver

Chapter 18

Sleep Essentials

One of the biggest questions exhausted new parents have is: when will my baby sleep through the night? The simple answer: by two months old, most newborns are sleeping six to eight hours straight. If your baby isn't, don't worry. There's a wide range of normal in child development.

Some lucky parents have those picture-perfect babies who do everything the guide books tell you to expect. Most parents experience roller-coaster "normal" sleep patterns through the first four months at least. Good nights on, and good nights off.

How well and how soon your baby sleeps through the night depends on many variables: weight gain, health, digestion, temperament (some babies are naturally night owls), home environment (stressed parents have stressed babies), and sleep environment (noise, lights, feeling safe). For most babies, by four months old, night waking is usually about comfort seeking, not hunger. Here are a few tips to help you manage your infant's sleep strategy.

Sleep Environment

Melatonin, which the body produces naturally and is essential to sleep, can only be produced in darkness. Sleep experts recommend a very dark room for better sleep patterns, and black out curtains—especially if street lights glare through your windows. As you are up with baby so much, you'll need a night light to navigate. Make sure the light is dim, not bright. The only type of light that does not disrupt melatonin production is red light.

White noise can help your baby sleep better, especially if you need to disguise street sounds. We used a sound machine with a timer that had soothing ocean waves, and set it for the first half hour of bedtime, then it automatically shut off.

Seven Tips for Sleep Success

1. Set up a few relaxing evening activities that signal to your baby she is going to bed: a bath, bedtime stories, soft music, gentle lights. Do the same relaxation routine every night, so your baby will recognize it's time to wind down.

2. Put baby to bed at the same time every night.

3. From birth to four months, most babies sleep better when swaddled. It lessens the chance they may wake themselves up, due to the startle reflex (jolting arms and legs), which tapers off around four months.

4. Teach your baby to fall asleep independently instead of in your arms. This leads to longer stretches of sleep. If the baby does fall asleep in your arms, gently wake him and then put him down in the crib.

5. If your baby wakes in the middle of the night, do not engage—just feed, burp and put him right back down. If you engage, the baby is likely to engage back—which is cute, but will quickly develop into an exhausting routine. Otherwise you'll be training your baby that midnight is playtime.

6. Don't change your baby at night, unless he has pooped or the diaper is so wet it's bothering him—which usually doesn't happen unless the baby has a diaper rash. Be sure to use nighttime diapers, which hold more wetness, and have a barrier protection to keep urine away from skin.

7. If your baby is gassy, add gripe water to his last feeding to reduce gas at night.

Sleep Transitions and Timing

After three weeks, Alessio had regained his birth weight and the doctor said we no longer needed to wake him at night to nurse. We could just feed him whenever he woke up. He was naturally waking up about 3 a.m. after sleeping a 6-7 hour stretch. Still, an improvement over the every 2.5 hours round-the-clock feeding marathon we'd been through since his birth. If I got to bed early enough, I could squeeze in six hours of sleep myself—which seemed like a three-week vacation to my sleep-starved body.

For the first six months, the baby should sleep in the same room with his parent(s). That's when babies are at highest risk of SIDS. According to sleep clinic studies, when babies hear the motions and breathing of the parent, it prevents them from falling into too deep a sleep and forgetting to breathe. For safety reasons, letting your baby sleep in bed with you is not recommended.

Once the baby moves into her own room after six months, it will take you and your baby several weeks to adjust to the transition. You will probably still be waking up just to check on your baby, and your baby will initially miss the natural sounds of your breathing and presence in the room. She might need a gentle pat or two in the middle of the night. Be patient.

A baby monitor is crucial for obvious safety reasons. It's also a device that comforts anxious parents. Many parents use a baby monitor for the first two years. Some are speakers only, which allow you to listen in to breathing or cries. I preferred one that had a camera, so I could actually see the baby sleeping.

For most babies, it's best to start the nighttime wind down between 5:30 and 6:30 p.m. (their natural down time). If you rev them up past the drowsy hour, they'll get their second wind. Though a laughing, engaged baby has her charms, so does Finally It's Mommy's Time, which hopefully is part of your night routine too.

> Keeping your baby up past her normal drowsy hour might give her a second wind.

When trying to adjust your baby to a longer night sleep routine, try to skip the middle-of-the-night feedings and let them whimper a bit. If your baby is crying, be there for him. You are still developing a bond of trust, and it's more helpful for your baby to know you are there and can be counted on, than to rigidly expect a baby to cry it out.

A big part of good parenting is finding the balance. You don't have to over-respond to every whimper, but if your baby is really crying and getting upset, don't ignore his signals or emotional needs. The best method is to gently enter the room, check to see that everything is okay, say a few soothing words, and give a soft reassuring touch. Let him settle a bit, then leave the room. Consistency is the key. It may take a few tries for you both, but you'll get there.

My pediatrician recommended sleep training at four months or at fourteen pounds. Dr. Raker's advice: if the baby wakes up in the middle of the night fussing, let him fuss in intervals of 5, 10, 15, and 20 minutes. This means to wait 5 minutes before going to comfort him. Once you have soothed him, remove yourself from being near the crib. If he is still fussing, wait 10 minutes before going back. Still fussing? Wait 15 minutes before giving a soothe, and on up to 20. This teaches gradual self-soothing, while letting the baby know you are near. It worked liked a charm. After three nights of sleep training, Alessio was sleeping for twelve hours straight! Hope it works as well for you.

Make It Easy on Yourself

Forget trying to think in the midnight haze. Who wants to *really* wake up as you stumble through the house, searching for a bottle, a timer, a burp rag? Thinking ahead is better than thinking in a daze.

- Before going to bed, set up your night feeding basics on your nightstand: bottle, burp cloth, formula, pacifier, tissues, night light or small flash light.

- Have extra pajamas and swaddle ready, in case baby wakes up soaked or soiled.

- If you are pumping at night, set up the necessary tools so you are pump ready for the feeding and can auto pilot through most of it (I call it REM feeding): pump and jump back into bed, and maybe even pick up that dream where you left off.

- If you need to warm milk and are using a bottle warmer, set it up so that all you have to do is place the bottle in the warmer and turn it on.

Crib Safety

Always put your child to sleep on his/her back to reduce the risk of sudden infant death syndrome (SIDS). Use a firm mattress. Crib bumpers are now considered unsafe by many SIDS organizations and child-safety advocates, including the American Academy of Pediatrics. "Bare is best," but if you decide to use bumpers, make sure they are breathable fabric and are properly and tightly affixed to the crib. Keep soft bedding, pillows and stuffed animals out of the crib for the first year. Use a sleep sack instead of a blanket. Never place a crib near a window or drapes, because your baby can become entangled in the blinds or curtain cords. Make sure all crib locks, latches and screws are tight and secure. For more on crib safety and guidelines, go to the Consumer Product Safety Commission at www.cpsc.gov.

Sleeping Essentials

☐ Crib & Mattress

- Slats do not exceed 2 3/8"
- No drop-side frames
- Converts into toddler bed. Saves $ in the long run.
- Organic mattress; or use BabeSafe cover on standard mattress.

☐ Crib Sheets

- Natural fabric sheets: cotton/bamboo
- Organics are best, made without dyes or pesticides that can irritate a baby's sensitive skin.

☐ Mobile & Sound Machine

- Soothing sights & sounds so senses are not overwhelmed
- Remote controlled mobile
- Automatic shut-off

☐ Pajamas

- Zip up or layette gown style (buy 3 total)
- Long & short sleeves, full coverage for legs/arms

☐ Swaddles

- Breathable natural fabrics: cotton/bamboo (buy 3 total)
- Use a swaddle with Velcro as a 2nd swaddle if your baby has Houdini-like powers.

☐ Sleep Sack

- Use when baby is no longer swaddled (about 4 months old).
- Lightweight & heavyweight for year-round comfort
- Use until age 2 or so.

$ = Money Saver

Chapter 19

Your Pediatrician and You

A good pediatrician is a must. After all, this person will be one of the most important advisors you'll have in navigating your children's health and well-being. It's important to have a single doctor giving advice who knows your child's medical history, including allergies, reactions, and sensitivities. If you do the shop-around approach, a little here and a little there, first one clinic, then another—you will likely get spotty advice and possibly incorrect treatment, as the clinic doctor won't have the full medical history on hand.

When choosing a pediatrician, consider the following: do you like and trust the doctor? Interview and ask tough questions. Make sure you and your doctor have similar viewpoints on the most important questions. What are those?

- Is your doctor comfortable and supportive with your viewpoints on how you wish to care for your children? (Whether your approach is holistic, traditional Western or integrative—a blend of both.)

- Does your doctor take the time to listen to your concerns, discuss options, and inform you to your satisfaction?

- Is your doctor available by phone, off-hours or on weekends? Who is her/his backup?

What to Expect on Your First Office Visit

Your newborn's first office checkup is usually at two weeks of age. The pediatrician will measure your baby's weight, length, and head size. She will also chart projected growth, so you'll get a sense of healthy development. She will perform a physical exam, and check your baby's reflexes, ability to focus, response to sounds, and general movements. The doctor's questions will involve your newborn's favorite activities: eating, peeing/pooping and sleeping. Setting up a vaccination schedule will also be an important part of your baby's first visit.

The average visit with a pediatrician is 15 minutes to ½ hour. During that time, your head is swimming. You'll forget a lot of the discussion, and if you don't come prepared (knowing what you want to ask), the time can fly by. To make the most of your appointment:

- Arrive prepared, notebook in hand. Inside your notebook should be your list of questions that have been accumulating since you got home from hospital. Write them down ahead of time as concerns come up. No question is silly or wrong. Don't feel embarrassed about your need to know, even if you are just curious about how things work.

- Take notes. Refer to them later, as needed. Track the vitals. Most doctors will give you a printout of weight, height, etc.

- Speak up and trust your intuition if you have any concerns about the doctor's recommendations, or need to further discuss a point—even if the doctor's clock has stopped ticking on your golden 15-minutes.

- It's important to develop a sense of trust with your pediatrician. If you don't feel right about your doctor or her practice, it's okay to switch to a better fit that works for you, your baby and family.

The Vaccination Question

Kids in the U.S. today get 55 doses of vaccines before they turn six. Are so many vaccines necessary? Which ones are? Who knows? That is why most parents opt to go the whole route of vaccinations recommended by the American Academy of Pediatrics (AAP).

I grew up in Spain, where only minimal vaccinations were required. My siblings and I actually had measles, mumps, chicken pox and so now have a life-long immunity to them, which vaccinations don't ensure. I also had whooping cough—which you *never* want your child to get.

Vaccines contain weakened forms of the diseases they are trying to prevent, along with adjuvants which deliberately cause inflammation, in order to stimulate your child's immune system so the vaccine will have a stronger effect. Many adjuvants also contain mercury or aluminum, which are toxins. Vaccines without mercury are available. Ask your doctor to prescribe these for your child.

I have friends who opted to not give their children any vaccines and go the holistic route. Other friends chose the full spectrum of vaccinations in line with AAP recommendations—no questions asked. Adriano and I are moderately in the middle. We chose to give our children all their vaccinations, but to vary the schedule so the babies weren't inundated by multiple shots at one time.

Dr. Oz recommends parents follow the AAP vaccination schedule. His reasoning: he's fine with parents taking a hand in adjusting the vaccination schedule, but most parents are busy and tend to forget the complicated, lengthy schedule (55 doses over 6 years). By following the AAP vaccination schedule, your doctor's office will remind you when your baby's shots are due and nothing gets confused or overlooked.

As parents, the choice is yours, but this important and complex choice is best made in conjunction with your doctor. Make sure you are well informed about the risks and benefits involved on both sides of the vaccination question. Familiarize yourself with the standard immunization schedule. Depending on your child's health, allergies, etc., your doctor may recommend variations to suit your child's needs.

Best Sites on Children's Health

So you love Google, especially parents with our 1001 questions. But there is a lot of incorrect information on the Internet. The best, most reliable sites for children's health info are:

- mayoclinic.org
- healthychildren.org
- kidshealth.org

Chapter 20

Watching Your Child Grow

Your child's first year is a time of firsts. The most rapid development and growth in a lifetime. Get ready to dance, because your baby is going to keep you on your feet! Keep in mind that all children develop at varying rates. Don't get alarmed (as I did) if your baby doesn't roll over from tummy to back at the five-month marker. Most children will be ahead on some markers, and behind on others. As long as the vitals are healthy, relax and enjoy watching your child grow.

What You Can Expect

BIRTH TO 3 MONTHS

Your newborn's wobbly head will soon find its strength. Neck muscles improve, especially with daily tummy time. (Lay your baby on her tummy on a comfortable mat; encourage her to lift head and shoulders.) Vision gets clearer and he is able to focus—especially on Mama's face during feedings.

- Between 6-8 weeks, you might see your baby's first smile! This is an infant's first social skill, and a sign of emotional growth—starting to display happiness in response to your smile.

- Over the next weeks, your baby may blow a few bubbles or make sounds of delight (gurgles and coo's) when you play with her.

- Babies will learn to reach toward you, and may grasp objects tightly for a few seconds. They are working on their hand-eye coordination, so you may catch them studying their hands.

- Between 2-3 months, baby's tummy time stretching and kicking may turn into partial rolls from side to back.

- Three months is a growth spurt, so your baby may be hungrier. Let her nurse as much as she wants. An added bonus for moms: nursing burns calories.

Parent Tips

Talk to your baby, hold kiss and snuggle, rock sing and laugh. Answer his cries. This baby is a gift—no matter how much he poops. Language is forming with every word your baby hears. Name things as you walk through the house or go on strolls. Use simple, everyday words to describe sights, sounds and smells. Stand in front of the mirror with your baby. Say "Mama" and your baby's name as you point. Your baby is soaking in the world around her, and though she has no words yet to express this, she is watching you for her cues.

Learning Through Play

* Newborns like to gaze. Offer your baby toys to look at. Introduce one at a time; allow your child to explore and focus on each one. Use a variety of shapes, sizes, and colors.

* Hold brightly colored toys over her chest as she lies on her back. She'll love reaching and pulling them close. Good toys at this age include rattles, a soft doll, or picture book.

* Infants like gentle sounds. A bright mobile with soft music or nature sounds can keep your baby both soothed and engaged.

4-6 MONTHS

Your baby becomes more aware of his surroundings and wants to explore. Most babies will be able to raise their heads while on their tummies (it's important to keep up the daily tummy time). Arms pump, legs kick as if baby is swimming in air. Wiggles get stronger. Your baby may learn to roll over, from back to front—which means you have to keep a hawk's eye on her when she is on the changing table or any high surface. As hand-eye coordination gets better, your baby will be able to purposely grasp objects and find ways to taste the world—everything goes into his mouth.

Your hawk's eye has to get even sharper in keeping choking materials out of his way. Do another safety inspection of your house, with special emphasis on small round items that your baby will magically be drawn to, and will be able to find, even though his vision has only recently learned to focus. (Use the toilet roll rule: if something is small enough to fit into a toilet roll, it's small enough for a child's windpipe.)

Look forward to your baby's first laugh and squeals—especially when you tickle her tummy. Little hands clapping. A magical time.

- Babies discover their body parts—tugging on ears is especially satisfying.

- First tooth may appear!

- Around 4 months, your baby will begin to recognize her own name.

- Around 5 months, your baby may learn to roll over or give a first hug.

- Around 6 months, your baby may sit up with assistance.

Parent Tips

Your baby may try to begin to talk—just burbles and a moment of waiting, to see if you will respond. Of course, you must talk back. In burble language if you want. Babies at this age respond to the emotional tone of a loving voice more than the actual words. They also like the goofy faces you make while imitating their babble. Baby talk is good for your baby's developing verbal skills, and babies love it —a language especially for them.

Learning Through Play

∗ Have fun. Play games. Peek-a-Boo, I See You teaches object permanence (that you are there, even when you are hidden behind something).

∗ Name the parts of the body. Counting toes. Kissing fingers. Arms, hands, nose. Babies love repetition. It is how they learn.

∗ Talk to your child about what you are doing. "I am getting your bottle ready" or "You are playing with your yellow car." This helps baby start to associate words with actions and objects, and develops vocabulary.

∗ Baby will start to imitate you. Shake a toy, then give it to him. Wait for him to respond. See if he tries to shake it too.

∗ Read to your baby, sing songs, lullabies and nursery rhymes. As early as four months, babies recognize the melodic rhythms of speech—an important part of language development.

7-9 MONTHS

Your baby will respond to her name, and will know yours too, saying *mama* or *dada*, along with more burbling attempts at conversation. Ask your baby questions, wait a moment, and see if your baby answers back. Your baby will be a real rock-and-roller, able to turn over in both directions, sit up, scoot, maybe even crawl or stand. Self-feeding begins. Experimenting with food, spoons, sippy cups, drool, tossing smearing finger-painting life. Creative pursuits include banging on Tupperware, a few sing-songy sounds that might be the start of a vocal career, playing some chords on the old Playskool piano—your baby is finding her genius. Natural talent is often displayed through a child's emerging interests. Watch your child for cues. Let him set the pace.

● Around 7-8 months, baby will have developed enough balance and strength to sit up in short stretches.

● Around 8-9 months, baby may start to scoot or crawl.

● Around 9 months, baby may be able to pull up to stand, using objects like a sofa or coffee table for support. This quickly leads to taking steps, cruising along the sofa's edge.

● Around 8-9 months, stranger anxiety may begin. Your baby may suddenly become shy or wary of strangers (including familiar friends and family). Don't pressure your baby to be social. Instead, be reassuring and give baby her space. Reassure loved ones (like grandparents), who might be hurt by the rejection. Give them tips on how best to approach your baby. A little bartering of toys and a gentle approach can work wonders. Stranger anxiety is a passing phase that peaks between 12-15 months, and goes down from there.

Parent Tips

Once your baby starts crawling, it's time for yet another safety inspection of your house. Things you thought were safe will suddenly loom out of the shadows, as you begin to recognize your baby's amazing and rapidly growing mobility. Take a walk on your hands and knees to better identify possible dangers.

Cover electric outlets, sharp corners on furniture; secure cabinets and drawers with safety-locks; move plants, floor lamps, toss anything you used to think was a nice decoration but that now could fall on your baby's head as she reaches, grabs and tries to pull herself up. You'll be tempted to make your house into a padded cell, for the time being.

When your baby begins to crawl, it's time for another safety check to baby-proof your home.

For a complete Checklist, see the "Home Safety Checklist" on page 166.

Your baby may also be able to pull to standing, which means the crib mattress must be moved to its lowest level. Remove bumpers or anything the child could use to climb out of bed.

Learning Through Play

＊ Your baby might enjoy stacking blocks and knocking them down.

＊ Play hide and seek. Be obvious. Hide behind the sofa, but leave your hand in plain view. Coax your baby to "find" you.

 ✳   Read to your baby every day. Place books in baby's reach.

 ✳   Get a few toys with buttons that make sounds or perform an action. Let your baby push the button on a musical toy, for instance, then dance to the music. This teaches cause and effect, and builds baby's confidence that she can make things happen.

 ✳   Creativity begins to blossom. Let your baby finger-paint with mashed pumpkin or applesauce on the highchair tray. (No paints yet, as baby will try to eat them.)

10-12 MONTHS

Your baby is getting stronger and more independent. Sitting on her own. Crawling all over the house. Taking the first step. An amazing cognitive transformation takes place—your baby knows when you are out of the room or hiding. All those peek-a-boo games have paid off. A little monkey, your child will imitate you (this can be both hilarious and scary). My baby destroyed my sister's cell phone, trying to talk like his dad. So we got him a play one, which suited him fine. He had many friends, of course, that he had long conversations with in delightful babble, just like his dad.

When you ask your baby to say *bye-bye*, she might wave back, blow kisses or shake her head No! Music is a language too and babies respond by singing clapping and tapping toes to the rhythm of a beat. The dance continues, and your baby continues to grow.

 •   Language skills develop rapidly. Your child will respond to simple requests. You may hear exclamations like *Whoa!* or *Uh-oh!*

 •   By twelve months, babies usually take their first steps without support, which quickly leads to walking.

 •   Once walking, your child will use both hands more freely to gather up toys and carry them around, bringing you gifts and objects of interest. Be sure to say "thank you" and take a moment to appreciate your child's efforts.

Parent Tips

When does discipline begin? As early as eight months, babies learn the words *yes* and *no*. Unfortunately parents use *No* more often (seven times more) than *Yes*, and the more you use it, the less effective it is.

So how do you get to *Yes* with your child? One way is to "catch" her when she is being good and praise her for it! Ignore or distract unwanted behavior. Direct attention to solutions by saying things like, "Let's try this." If your baby wants to play with an electric plug, say a firm, "No." Follow up with, "That's not a toy. Let's go play with your toys."

Learning Through Play

* Rolling a ball back and forth teaches hand-eye coordination, along with a few physics lessons on aim and force. How hard or soft your baby pushes affects the distance the ball will go. Does your baby's aim improve the more you play this game?

* Go exploring in your backyard. Find bugs, flowers, birds. Touch tree bark. Crinkle leaves in your fingers. Smell flowers. Name colors. Teach your child to explore his senses.

* Take a sound walk around the neighborhood, listening for trucks, motorcycles, birds, cats. Name and imitate the sounds.

* Pretend play is a good way to build your child's imagination and intelligence. Put out a few objects like an empty cup or a plastic plate and spoon. Pretend you are eating or drinking and see if your child will do the same. Games like this help develop language ability because it enhances symbolic thinking, which is the base for all language learning. It also teaches the child about ideas and how to transform the everyday world, which is the basis for all the arts and sciences.

As Albert Einstein said, "Imagination is more important than knowledge. For knowledge is limited to all we now know and understand, while imagination embraces the entire world, and all there ever will be to know and understand."

Growing With Your Child

Life is about attitude, and so is parenting. I can list the milestones and check them off, but the finer points of raising a child are more complex. Every step your child takes, you will take one too. A good parent responds, engages, and encourages their children along. It really *is* a dance. Every new stage of development offers excitement, pleasure and reward for both you and your child. Here are a few lessons I've learned about the emotional milestones in life.

Confidence

When I was growing up, through all the trials and triumphs of childhood, I knew I could depend on two things: the unconditional love of my family, and the fact that we could laugh at almost anything. Confidence and laughter go together. It's when we take things too seriously, that we can't see our way out.

Whether I won or lost, my family always told me that I was great, beautiful, and smart—all the things I didn't quite feel, but hoped were true. They were sowing seeds of confidence for the future me— the woman I would become. That's what we need to give our kids at any age, whether baby, toddler, adolescent or teen. Love. Listening. Encouragement. These are the building blocks of self-confidence.

Confidence is linked to health, happiness, and success in every area of life. What is confidence anyway? For me, it's the courage to keep trying, to not be afraid of failure. As Professor Cornel West of Princeton once said, "Of course it's a failure, but how good of a failure is it?"

People who lack confidence are afraid to make mistakes. Therefore they learn less, because it's the mistakes that teach us the most. Really, let's drop that word, *mistake*. Let's think: Explore. Grow. Learn.

Children are naturally born with confidence. How many times do they fall before they learn to run? How many words do they garble before the language flows? Take a walk with a toddler. Every two minutes he stops to touch a flower, examine an ant carrying a leaf, watch a leaf sailing down the gutter after a rain, taste a stick, roll on the grass. What confidence! Can you imagine if adults dared to do the same?

Children are learning all the time—especially from the words we use. Whether praise or criticism, they take it to heart. Rather than just praise your children for what they accomplish, praise them for who they are. Encourage their natural curiosity. Emphasize process over outcomes. Practice positive speaking until it is a habit. Put yourself in your child's shoes, and ask yourself, "How would I want to be treated?"

If you've been negative in the past, it takes confidence and a conscious effort to change. Here are some empowering phrases to sprinkle into your vocabulary: *You can do it! You're amazing! Keep trying!*

I say those phrases to my kids, but also to myself. It takes courage to be a good parent. One of the hardest and most rewarding jobs on the planet. Just remember: *You're amazing! Keep trying! You can do it!*

Chapter 21

Going Back To Work

I felt excited, slightly guilty, and a little scared. It was my first day back at work after three months of maternity leave, blissfully inundated with my newborn Sienna, and my toddler Alessio, who was nearly two.

I couldn't seem to find my "professional" persona. Maybe she was still asleep. Maybe I had lost her altogether. The adult world seemed far off, a little chaotic, as I put aside my fears and picked up my son.

Then worry stepped in, as if that was my real job as a mother: WORRY all in caps—about every eventuality, which I had tried to cover in my numerous spreadsheets papering the fridge, ensuring the house would run smoothly while I was at work. *Babies fed like clockwork, nutritional menus for the week, shopping lists, emergency phone numbers, and what else?* I couldn't remember.

I tried to let it go, shift gears into the professional adult me—the woman that people looked to for answers, to questions other than those I'd been answering the past few months: *Do you know where the pacifier is? Are we out of diapers? Where the bleep is the Mylicon!?*

As I put on my makeup, I explained to Alessio that Mama was going to "work." He remembered that word and frowned.

Alessio came with me to the car and watched me drive down the street. My sister Marisa, aka Aunt Riri, was holding him. I kept waving until I couldn't see Alessio anymore, and he did the same. I felt torn in two. I ached to leave him so sweetly, so plainly missing me, while I swallowed a double-dollop of guilt. I actually *wanted* to go back to work. I missed my old identity, recognition in the adult world. A professional. Wearing high heels and silk blouses instead of burp rags.

While driving, I noticed some spit up on my blouse. "Badge of honor," I said to myself, thinking about a recent TED talk by Brené Brown, a research professor who has studied vulnerability for over a decade. Dr. Brown said vulnerability was at the core of shame, fear and struggle for worthiness, but it was also the birthplace of joy, creativity, belonging and love. "Fully embrace vulnerability," she said. "What makes you vulnerable also makes you beautiful."

> Sometimes doing "our best" means to stop all the running around and be in the moment.

I arrived at work a bit discombobulated, but glad to see everyone. Around the water cooler, co-workers caught me up on all the office stories. I was laughing so hard my cheeks hurt. My stories were all about my kids. The return to the adult world felt strange, like I had a very long umbilical cord attached to my other life as Mom.

There was a bit of chaos when I got home. My kids (husband included) were vying for my attention and I wished I could stretch myself like Elastigirl from *The Incredibles* and give everybody exactly what they needed. But I couldn't.

Most moms are 110-percenters. We try to give our children our best. But what does 110 percent actually mean? We are giving more than we've got. Sometimes "our best" is to stop all the running around and be in the moment.

I took a deep breath and thought, "It's okay to be imperfect and let things get under my skin. It's okay to be this muddled," as I zoned in on the kids and shifted gears yet again that day. And with this gentle permission to be myself, no more, no less, I began to relax and even enjoy the beautiful imperfections of life.

Crunched for Time?

- Give yourself a 15 minute buffer in the morning. Benefits: peace of mind, no smeared eyeliner, and your kids won't feel like ping-pong balls as you rush to feed them, brush their teeth, get them dressed, etc.

- When you are overloaded, stop and regroup. Ask yourself: is this the best use of my time right now?

- If you feel that you are always rushing, rearrange your schedule or trim it down.

- Make time each day to recharge. You are just as important as your kids. What you don't do today, will be there tomorrow. Sometimes it's best to delay your chores and refresh your soul.

Practical Tips on Returning to Work

Prepare yourself and your child, and your caregiver, by doing some trial runs a few days before you go back to work. Give your baby a big kiss and hug, and say, "I'll be back soon." If your baby consistently has trouble with you leaving, work out a plan with your caregiver on the best way to distract him.

At work, be firm about quitting time. Leave work at the same time each day—no matter what is left to do, the work can (and will) be waiting for you the next day.

Pumping at work: arrange a private space, if possible. Be sure your boss/colleagues are aware of your schedule, so that you won't be interrupted. If you don't have a private space, consider hanging a sign on the bathroom door: *Pumping in Progress: Please don't disturb.* Don't feel bad knowing that everyone outside the bathroom can hear the machine's swooshing sound, and you're picturing them picturing you attached to the suction cups. I took my iPhone into the bathroom, so that I could look at my baby, in hopes that I would pump more milk.

At home, be firm about spending time with your children. No matter what chaos might be waiting, my first hour home is time with the kids. You might be tired, but make it a point to connect and enjoy your time with family.

If you have more than one child, make sure you have time together as a family, and time alone with each child. The alone time should be as free from disruption as possible. In adjusting to change, older children generally need more reassurance than infants. My pediatrician told me to put my infant Sienna down an hour before Alessio, my toddler, went to bed. That way he would have my undivided attention each day, and it would lessen any jealousy he might feel toward his little sister. It worked!

Setting Up Serenity: Childcare Options

Finding the right caretakers for your children will ease the stress of going back to work. Depending upon your budget, there are a variety of options.

- Full-time nanny: Gives your child the most personal attention, but also costs the most. Pay scale and benefits vary based on where you live. Usually professional nannies expect paid holidays and one-week vacation a year.

- Share a nanny with another family: Considerably cuts down care costs, while giving your child more personal attention than traditional daycare.

- Drop off with stay-at-home mom: This can work well, especially if she lives nearby and you know her. If not, make sure she has good references. A key factor in choosing this option is the number of kids the mom is caring for, which directly affects how much personal attention your child will receive.

- Grandparents nearby can be a great arrangement.

- Traditional daycare: It's best to find a small nursery with high adult-to-child ratio. Get references from other parents. Be sure to find out the drop-off and pick-up times and policy, and that they meet your schedule needs. What is the general atmosphere?
  - Does the staff engage with babies in their care?
  - Do the children look happy and well cared for?
  - Is the place clean (including shared toys) and well organized?
  - What kind of toys and activities are available?

Choosing a Nanny

Finding a good nanny or childcare provider can come from a variety of sources. Friends and other moms are the best resource. The basic questions are experience, availability (does their schedule work with your needs?), and references. If you plan on the caretaker driving your child anywhere, he or she will need a valid drivers license and insurance. (Be sure to get a copy, once hired.) CPR training is a definite asset. Low-cost classes are available in most communities via Red Cross or other organizations. It's advisable to do a background check and Google the person's name.

The Interview

My friend, Carolina, gave me this list of eight good questions to ask potential nannies:

1 How long was your longest nanny position?

2 What was your shortest nanny position and why?

3 Do your current employers know that you are looking for another position? Would they give you a reference? (Don't accept references from family members.)

4 Do you have any formal childhood development training? Describe the age groups you have worked with, and what you like about them.

5 What has been the most challenging thing about working with other people's children?

6 What do you like best about being a nanny?

7 What are you looking for in your next position? What is the desired pay? Do you have school or other activities that may require specific time off during the day?

8 Pose a scenario about discipline, an emergency, or something else that might concern you. Her response will give you insight into her decision-making process and views on raising children.

How do you know if the person will be compatible with your family? Go with your gut. Let the baby interview too. See how the caretaker holds him, what rapport they have. This is more important than if she knows how to change a diaper—all of that can be taught. Interaction and communication with a child are instinctual. I want someone who talks to my baby, will sing and dance with him—naturally, not because she is told to, or pretends to only when I'm around. I want someone who smiles at the baby, and the baby smiles back.

In short, the qualities I am looking for with in-home help are: heart, common sense, honesty and trustworthiness, a happy disposition, and great references.

I've been through four childcare providers with my two children. Wonderful Elena has three grown children of her own. Selena was a grandmother of five. I wanted women with experience, and not just experience, but heart. They cuddled and cooed my babies, and Sienna and Alessio were as comfortable with them as with anyone in my family. In fact, they were family. What else do you call someone who is so intimately helping you raise your child?

Childcare providers will come and go, most of them for their own personal reasons. Out of four home helpers, only one was a problem and I had to let her go. If you feel uncomfortable with someone you've hired or how your baby is behaving (crying more often, whiny, sad), trust your instincts and ask questions. It doesn't hurt to come home early and surprise your sitter just to see how things are really going.

My current childcare arrangement is a combination of part-time helpers, family included: Elena; my husband, Adriano; and my sister, Marisa. Between the four of us, we get everything done and the kids are happy.

Quick & Easy: Tips for Going Back to Work

1   Create a weekly meal plan and make some freezer meals ahead of time. Planning and preparation will lead to smoother evenings after a long day at work.

2   Lay out everything the night before: your clothes, the baby's clothes, a re-stocked diaper bag, pack your lunch, wash your pump parts and have it packed and ready to go for the next day. Do everything you can to make your mornings easier for you and baby.

3   Consider showering at night to buy yourself extra time in the mornings.

4   Create a weekly cleaning schedule that allows you to do small chores daily in 20-minute time-spans. Helps you stay sane, as you won't have to spend weekends or evenings frantically trying to keep up with the housework. If you are able to hire a cleaning service to help on a weekly or monthly basis, do it!

5   Do a trial run at daycare the week before you return to work. It will give the baby some time to adjust, and will help you to better establish your morning routine before your actual return.

6   Going back to work after having a baby is HARD. Leaving your baby for the first time is an emotional experience, no matter how much you love your job. It is okay to feel upset. But do know that it gets easier as time goes on, and you won't always feel this way.

Chapter 22

Super Mom Shuffle

In every ending there is a beginning, and so it seems appropriate to end this book with the first blog I ever wrote. *(Reprinted from www.princessivana.com)*

When I was a kid growing up in Spain, my brother, sister and I used to write and perform skits. It was during the days of the Rambo movies. We created a character called Ramba, Super Mom. Ramba could do a thousand things at once—ironing a ceiling-high stack of clothes while making dinner, changing diapers, super shopping (3,000 items on her list) and all with a sparkling clean house. She was drying tears and singing an opera, dancing through her thousands of chores—and she might as well have been wearing a crown and maybe some glass slippers, too, for how much we loved that fairy tale of Ramba, Super Mom!

Now I'm a mom and have updated my version of Ramba. My thousand things include high-level negotiations with a toddler at home and executives at work. Sometimes I want to burp my boss and take notes from my newborn! I call it the Super Mom Shuffle.

Can we really have it all? What does it even mean these days?

So I'm working on giving my kids confidence, and teaching them to dream big like my parents taught me. For my baby, Sienna, teaching her confidence means being there when she cries, or hopefully *before* she cries by reading her body language—the way she puckers or roots, the way her hands flail the air, her feet pumping like she's on a bike. For my toddler, Alessio, it is about taking the time to listen to him (even though he doesn't quite know yet what he is trying to say) and helping him find the words.

All of life is about communication and paying attention to the signals, whether they are your child's or your own needs which so often get lost in the Super Mom Shuffle. My mother had an opera she sang when she was about to explode. *Opera of the Mad Housewife*, she jokingly called it. The lyrics varied from situation to situation, and rather than curse (which she sometimes did), she mostly sang. Sang her heart out, all her frustrations, sang them into some wild sound coming from her throat. The words often rhymed and all my friends agreed, she had a great voice.

So fellow mothers-in-arms (arms full of babies), let's break the paralyzing myth of motherly perfection by singing our own songs— whatever they may be. We get to write the music and lyrics, and even do our own dance. Let's not forget that!

I love kids and learning, and we all know kids are the best teachers around. My two-year-old son, Alessio, is learning the meaning of "happy." He knows what it is, though he can't speak a full sentence. He looks at his sister laughing and says, *Happy*. He looks at our family standing together in front of the mirror and says, *Happy*.

What does it mean to have it all? *This*, I think. *This moment in front of the mirror.*

So yes, I am a real princess and I could choose to raise my children by remote control, but I would be missing one of the most magical parts of my life.

Here's to mothers everywhere and to your happily ever after!

Reference

Quick Reference Section

Love It, Check It—The Ultimate Essentials

As I prepared for my first baby's shower, I thought about my sister-in-law, who had started crying when she logged on to Babies R' Us to register for her baby shower. She was driven into a temporary bout of brain freeze, overwhelmed by too many choices and no clear idea of what she actually needed. For my shower, I decided to e-mail my already-mommy girlfriends and ask them to name their top *must-haves* for newborns. Their recommendations were so helpful to me, I wanted to share them with you. I've also added in my own new mom *must-haves*.

The result is the Love It, Check It list, a simple two-page checklist of the ultimate essentials: my favorite products tried and true, along with all the practical necessities you and your baby will need in the first year (compiled from the Essentials Lists throughout the book). I want to make it easy. This is a comprehensive list that will save you time. One-stop shopping with Mom in mind.

Check out Love It, Check It on the next two pages. Hope you love it too.

Love It Check It

NURSERY

- ☐ Crib & Mattress
- ☐ Glider/Rocking Chair
- ☐ Baby Monitor
  - Summer Infant Day & Night
  - Philips Avent DECT Digital
- ☐ Changing Table, Pad & Covers
- ☐ Diaper Trashcan
  - Dekor Diaper Disposal System
- ☐ Swing
  - Fisher Price swings
- ☐ Stationary Exersaucer
  - Graco Baby Einstein
- ☐ Play Mat for Tummy Time
  - Skip*Hop Farmyard Play Mat
- ☐ Books
  - Dr. Seuss & Sandra Boynton books are my kids' faves.
- ☐ Toys
  - Rhino Toys Oball
  - Neurosmith Sunshine Symphony

BABY GEAR

- ☐ Car Seat
- ☐ Stroller
- ☐ Baby Carrier
  - Ergobaby Carrier
- ☐ Diaper Bag/Purse
  - Storksak Diaper Bag
- ☐ Feeding & Sleeping Timer
  - Itzbeen Baby Care Timer, Total Baby App

NEWBORN

- ☐ Onesies
  - Carter's, Chicco
- ☐ Tops & Bottoms
- ☐ Coats & Sweaters
- ☐ Socks & Shoes
  - Babysoy Socks
  - Stride Rite, Pediped
- ☐ Hats
- ☐ Blankets
  - Aden + Anais Muslin Lightweight Blankets
- ☐ Diaper & Changing
  - Pampers Swaddlers Sensitive Diapers
  - Huggies Pull-Ups Night Diapers
  - Balmex Diaper Rash Cream
  - Huggies Gentle Care Sensitive Baby Wipes
- ☐ Grooming: Nail file & clippers, toothbrush & hairbrush
- ☐ Lotion & Soap
  - California Baby Skincare Line
  - Aquaphor
  - Cetaphil
  - Cortaid (with 1% hydrocortisone)
- ☐ Infant Bathtub
  - 4moms Cleanwater Tub
- ☐ Hand Sanitizer

Love It ❤ Check It

FEEDING

- ☐ Breast Pump, Bra & Storage Bags
  - • Medela Pump in Style Breast Pump
  - • Simple Wishes Hands Free Breast Pump Bra
- ☐ Breast Feeding Relief
  - • Motherlove Nipple Cream
  - • Ameda ComfortGel Hydrogel Pads
- ☐ Breastfeeding Pillow
- ☐ Nursing Bra
  - • Bravado Nursing Bra
- ☐ Bottles
  - • Dr. Brown's Bottles & Nipples
- ☐ Bottle Drying Rack
- ☐ Bottle Warmer
- ☐ Formula
  - • Good Start Gentle Formula by Nestlé
- ☐ Solid Food
  - • Earth's Best Organic Baby Food
  - • Plum Organics Just Prunes
- ☐ Burp Cloths & Bibs
- ☐ Sippy Cups, Spoons, Forks & Bowls
  - • Nuk, Avent Magic & Thinkbaby Sippy Cups
- ☐ High Chair

FUSSY BABY

- ☐ Gas Relief
  - • Wellements Gripe Water (all natural)
  - • Mylicon Gas Relief
- ☐ Teething & Pacifier
  - • Boiron Camilia Teething Relief (all natural)
  - • Sophie the Giraffe Teether Toy
  - • Sassy Bee Teething Toys
  - • Baby Safe Teething Feeder by Sassy Baby
  - • The First Years Soothie Pacifier
- ☐ Anti-Allergy Medicine
- ☐ Cough & Cold: Nasal aspirator, fever reducer, thermometer & humidifier
  - • Little Noses Saline Spray
- ☐ The Happiest Baby on the Block DVD

SLEEPING

- ☐ Crib & Mattress
- ☐ Crib Sheets
- ☐ Mobile & Sound Machine
  - • Tiny Love Nature's Soothing Serenade Musical Mobile
- ☐ Pajamas
- ☐ Swaddles
  - • Baby's Own Swaddling Blanket
  - • SwaddleMe Adjustable Infant Wrap
  - • Sleep Sack

Home Safety Checklist

Although many of the following ideas won't apply until your baby becomes mobile, that time will sneak up on you. Here's a list for you to use over the next year to get ready for that day.

- ☐ Post the number of the Poison Control Center near your phone.

- ☐ What types of live plants do you have in your home? Know their names and contact the Poison Control Center to find out if they are safe or poisonous.

- ☐ Tie up your mini-blind cords to prevent possible strangulation.

- ☐ Block off all electrical outlets with inserts or furniture to prevent electric shock.

- ☐ Cushion the brick around your fireplace hearth if it is an area that will be available to your baby; remove pokers and other fireplace equipment.

- ☐ Make sure that all cribs and baby furniture or toys that could be chewed on have only lead-free paint.

- ☐ Install gates over stairway entrances and other hazardous areas of your house.

- ☐ Install cabinet locks for all cabinets that contain potentially harmful products. (The most effective cabinet locks are Tot-Loks®, a magnetic lock that won't allow the cabinet to be opened without the special magnet the parents keep up high.) The cheapest and most effective prevention is to remove harmful products from low cabinets. Keep them higher than a toddler can reach.

- ☐ Make sure furniture can't be tipped over when your baby starts pulling up. Secure chests of drawers to the wall.

- ☐ Remove all grocery store plastic bags and the like from areas that toddlers can reach.

☐ Install a toilet lid lock, or get into the habit of keeping the bathroom doors shut at all times.

☐ Remove flowing tablecloths that could be a hazard when your baby starts pulling up.

☐ Plan a fire safety escape route.

☐ Install fire alarms and carbon monoxide sensors.

☐ Cushion sharp edges of coffee tables and furniture.

☐ Adjust the thermostat on your water heater so that hot water can't come out above 120°, to prevent scaldings.

☐ Buy a thermometer or tub toy to check the baby's bath water. About 85° is recommended for a newborn's bath temperature.

☐ Check small toys for choking hazards by using the toilet paper roll test. If the toy can fit into a toilet paper roll, it can be swallowed, and possibly block a baby's airway.

☐ Plan to use stationary toys like Exersaucers® or other baby seats, rather than walkers.

☐ Visit your local fire or police station, or hospital to be sure you have your car seat properly installed.

☐ Remove all bedside medication, lotions, perfumes, etc. to a safe location.

Developmental Milestones: 1-15 Months

Milestones: 2 Weeks-1 Month

Look forward to your baby looking at you and following your face when you move. She will try to lift her head when she is on her tummy. She will also tell you what she wants by fussing and crying.

What You Can Do

Give your baby lots of attention. If he cries, comfort him. If he's hungry, feed him. You cannot spoil your baby at this age. Give your child tummy time for at least one minute each day.

Begin a routine at nighttime to teach your child that it's bedtime. Trying to get her to fall asleep "on her own"—instead of in your arms—will teach her to fall asleep independently. This will lead to longer stretches of sleep.

Safety Tips

Always put your child to sleep on his back to reduce the risk of sudden infant death syndrome (SIDS). No soft bedding or pillows.

Avoid crowded areas where your baby may be exposed to sick people.

Have everyone wash their hands or use Purell whenever they hold her.

Place your car seat in the back seat and rear facing.

Check that your water heater is set to less than 120 degrees; otherwise scalding can occur in seconds.

Helpful Hints

Gas and colic may cause your baby to be fussy. Try swaddling him, laying him on his side, rocking him gently (never shaking), or making a shhhh-ing sound. You can also try Mylicon drops, Hylands Colic Tabs, gripe water or chamomile tea.

When to Call the Doctor

If your baby has a temperature of 100.4°F degrees or higher, is feeding poorly, or looks yellow.

Milestones: 1-2 Months

Look forward to your baby looking at your face and smiling when you hold him. He will start to follow your face when you move and try to lift his head when he is on his tummy. He will also tell you what he wants by fussing or crying.

What You Can Do

Give your baby lots of attention. If she cries, comfort her. If she's hungry, feed her. You cannot spoil your baby at this age.

Give your child tummy time for a few minutes each day. Offer your baby objects to look at and touch. He can focus best when objects are 8-12 inches away. Play tracking games by moving your face and toys back and forth. Talk and sing to your baby and respond to him when he cries.

Begin a routine at nighttime to teach your child that it's bedtime. Trying to get him to fall asleep "on his own"—instead of in your arms—will teach him to fall asleep independently. This will lead to longer stretches of sleep.

Safety Tips

Always put your child to sleep on his back to reduce the risk of sudden infant death syndrome (SIDS). No soft bedding or pillows.

Avoid crowded areas where he may be exposed to sick people.

Place your car seat in the back and rear facing.

Check that your water heater is set to less than 120 degrees; otherwise, scalding burns can occur within seconds.

Helpful Hints

Gas and colic may cause your baby to be fussy. Try swaddling him, laying him on his side, rocking him gently (never shaking), or making a shhhh-ing sound. You can also try Mylicon drops, Hylands Colic Tabs, gripe water or chamomile tea.

When to Call the Doctor

If your baby has a temperature of 100.4°F degrees or higher, is feeding poorly, or looks yellow.

Milestones: 2-4 Months

Look forward to your baby cooing, smiling and laughing more. She may start to grab her own hands, put them in her mouth and drool a lot more. She will also be able to focus for longer periods of time and follow you as you walk across the room.

What You Can Do

Introduce one toy at a time and allow your child to explore and focus on each one.

Hold brightly colored toys over his chest as he lies on his back and he'll love reaching and pulling them close. Good toys at this age include rattles, a soft doll, or picture book.

Encourage tummy time to help build strong neck and back muscles.

Safety Tips

Always put your child to sleep on his back to reduce the risk of sudden infant death syndrome (SIDS). No soft bedding or pillows.

Your car seat should still be in the back and rear facing and used every time your child rides in a car until 2 years of age.

Always watch your baby in the bathtub. Drowning can happen very quickly even in shallow water, so take him with you if you need to leave the room.

Helpful Hints

Continue breast or formula feeding. She is still too young for solids and does not need any water or juice.

Good news! Colic will end soon. Gas and colic may cause your baby to be fussy. Try swaddling, laying him on his side, rocking him gently (never shaking), or making a shhh-ing sound. You can also try Mylicon drops, Hylands Colic Tabs, gripe water or chamomile tea.

Milestones: 4-5 Months

Look forward to your child rolling over more. He may stick his hands and feet in his mouth, drool more and grab his ears because it is comforting and he is finding these new body parts. He may start grabbing at objects and transferring them from one hand to the next. You may even see a little tooth pop through the gum line.

What You Can Do

Try placing your baby in different positions such as her back, tummy and in a sitting position with support. Let her play with your fingers and respond back when she coos and talks with you. Continue giving her tummy time.

Safety Tips

Your child is capable of rolling over. Never leave him unattended on a changing table, sofa or bed because he can roll off!

Always put your child to sleep on her back, but if she rolls to her stomach on her own, do not worry. Keep soft bedding and stuffed animals out of the crib for the first year.

Your car seat should still be in the back and rear facing and used every time your child rides in a car until 2 years of age.

Helpful Hints

Exersaucers and bouncers may be fun toys. Infant walkers are a no-no.

Your child may start watching you eat. She still gets all the nutrition she needs from breast milk or formula. You can begin giving solid foods at 4-6 months old.

Yes, colic is over! You deserve to sleep through the night and your child can now do it safely too. Nighttime waking is usually behavioral and due to comfort seeking, not hunger. It is safe to sleep train your child if you would like.

Milestones: 6-8 Months

Look forward to your child making sounds such as "bababa" and "dada." She will begin to be aware of an object's presence even when it is hidden. As a result, she will enjoy playing peek-a-boo. She may begin to sit up well and may start crawling and standing up with support.

What You Can Do

Continue an active dialogue with your child. Explain what you are doing, for example, "Yummm, you're eating applesauce."

Press a button or shake a toy and allow time for him to try. Give him time to respond and imitate your actions.

Provide a variety of safe toys and encourage exploration.

Start playing games like peek-a-boo.

Safety Tips

Your child will soon be mobile. This is an exciting time but a safety concern. Start safety-proofing your entire house. Things to think about include: poisons, medications, cleaning supplies and hazardous materials locked up high in cabinets; electric outlet covers; toilet seat cover locks; gates blocking all stairwells; window locks; tie curtain blind cords up high; cover or lock up small trash cans like the ones in the bathroom where you might throw away sharp objects such as a disposable razor or medications; get in the habit of placing all visitors' bags and purses on a high shelf.

Always have the number for Poison Control handy (1-800-222-1222).

Always have Children's Benadryl at home. You can use this if your child has an allergic reaction to food.

Helpful Hints

Yipee! Your little one is eating more solid foods.

She may begin crying when you put her down or leave a room. This is the beginning of separation anxiety. Comfort her as much as you can, but understand you may have to leave to run errands or go to work and she will be okay.

Milestones: 8-10 Months

Look forward to more cruising. Your child may start standing on her own and taking a few steps. She may start saying words like "mama," "dada," waving bye-bye, and blowing kisses. She will continue to try to feed herself.

What You Can Do

Comfort your child when he cries and acknowledge his feelings when he is frustrated.

Ask him questions like, "Do you want this toy?" and wait for him to respond and then give it to him. These conversations help develop his social, emotional, language and even motor skills.

Play hide-and-seek and encourage her participation in games like placing a block in its proper hold or building a tower.

Be reassuring when you leave her and tell her you will be back and that you will miss her.

Reassure him when he cries for you at night, but try not to pick him up or rock him back to sleep because this will make it difficult for him to learn to soothe himself back to sleep. It is normal for children who have previously slept through the night to wake up during the night.

Safety Tips

Keep small objects out of reach. Continue to look around the house for safety concerns. Safety proof your home, as children will get into everything at this age.

Crib mattresses should be moved to their lowest level once your child is pulling to stand. Remove all bumpers that can be used as an aid to climb out of the crib.

Continue to buckle up your child in the back car seat, rear facing.

Remember the number for Poison Control (1-800-222-1222).

Milestones: 8-10 Months, con't.

Helpful Hints

Try finger foods. Practice using a sippy cup.

Keep your child's new teeth healthy by cleaning them with a washcloth, finger-brush or soft toothbrush after feedings. Avoid giving the bottle in bed. This will cause cavities and increase ear infections.

Your child may start crying when friends or family come to visit even if he used to go to them without a problem. This is the beginning of stranger anxiety. Comfort your child and reassure your family and friends that everything is fine and he will outgrow this phase by 18 months of age.

Milestones: 10-12 Months

Look forward to more cruising and walking! Your child may start standing on her own and taking a few steps. She will likely have a few words like "mama" and "dada." She may be able to point to body parts and know a few animal sounds. She will continue to become more independent by self-feeding, and she may not want you to feed her.

What You Can Do

Comfort your child when he cries and acknowledge his feelings when he is frustrated. Ask him questions like "do you want this doll?" and wait for him to respond and then give it to him. These conversations help develop his social, emotional, language and even motor skills.

Play hide-and-seek and encourage participation in games like placing a block in its proper hole or building a tower.

Safety Tips

Keep small objects out of reach. Continue to inspect the house for safety concerns.

Make sure to buckle up your child in the back car seat, rear facing.

Remember the number for Poison Control (1-800-222-1222).

Helpful Hints

Your child may be able to drink out of a sippy cup.

Keep your child's new teeth healthy by cleaning them with a finger-brush or a soft toothbrush after feedings. Avoid giving a bottle in bed. This will cause cavities and increase ear infections.

Stranger anxiety may still occur. If your child doesn't want to go to others, comfort her and reassure your family and friends that everything is fine and she will outgrow this phase by 18 months of age.

Milestones: 12-15 Months

Look forward to your child speaking more. She may say 3-10 words by 15 months and begin to point and name some body parts. She will start to understand more and more and begin to follow simple directions. She may start stacking blocks 2 or 3 high. She may also begin to run and climb.

What You Can Do

Toddlers understand a lot more than they can say. Encourage your child to use his words to communicate. Read to your child and play games that involve pretending and imitating such as play kitchen or toy telephone. You should "narrate" your day, so he learns to put words to the things he is doing each day.

Safety Tips

Continue to safety proof your house so exploring is safe and fun. Be careful of bookshelves and stove tops that used to seem unreachable but are now accessible to your child's climbing. Keep small, hard objects out of reach.

Avoid nuts, gum, popcorn, hot dogs, whole grapes, whole carrots and hard candy until your child is 3 years old because they are choking risks.

Car seats should remain rear-facing until your child is 2, or outgrows the highest height or weight allowed by the car seat manufacturer.

Helpful Hints

You may switch from formula or breast milk to whole milk. Whole milk has a lot of fat that is good for brain development and 16-24oz/day provides an adequate amount of calcium. Continue to wean the bottle and encourage a cup. All foods at this age are OK from an allergy perspective.

Keep your child's vaccinations up to date. The vaccines are safe and will not cause developmental delay or autism.

Brush your child's teeth twice a day with a wet cloth or a soft toothbrush, with water or non-fluoridated baby toothpaste. Make it fun so he is not scared when he visits the dentist at 2 years of age.

Courtesy of Dr. Bess Raker, Beverly Hills Pediatrics

Feeding Chart for Baby's First Year

Feeding Chart: 0-4 Months

BREASTMILK	AMOUNT: At least 10-12 times within a 24-hour period. Every 2–2 ½ hours for the first couple of months. A baby should consume up to half his weight in ounces in a single feeding. If your baby weighs 8 pounds, offer him 4 ounces.
FORMULA	AMOUNT: At least 10-12 times within a 24-hour period. Every 2½ to 3 hours. INTAKE RANGE: 18–40 oz per day **Quick Tips** • When mixing formula, add the water first, then add formula and shake. • If you are feeding with a bottle, feed in the upright position. • Most newborns want to eat every 2-3 hours. Start with 1-2 oz at each feeding the first week, then work up to 2-4 oz. As your baby gets older and his tummy gets bigger, he'll drink fewer bottles a day with more formula in each. In a couple of months, he may be down to 6-8 bottles of 4-6 oz every 24 hours, depending upon your baby's intake range. • A baby should consume up to half his weight in ounces in a single feeding. If your baby weighs 8 pounds, offer him 4 ounces.
SOLIDS—None	No cereals, grains, fruits, vegetables, protein or dairy.

Feeding Chart: 4-6 Months

BREASTMILK	AMOUNT: At least 10-12 times within a 24-hour period. Every 2½ to 3 hours.
FORMULA	AMOUNT: At least 10-12 times within a 24-hour period. Every 2½ to 3 hours. INTAKE RANGE: 24-45 oz per day ### Quick Tips • Offer your baby 2.5 oz of formula per pound of body weight. • By 4 months, she'll probably drop to 4 or 5 bottles of 6-7 oz each. By 6 months, she'll typically be down to 3 or 4 bottles of 7-8 oz each a day.
SOLIDS	AMOUNT: .16 oz or 1 teaspoon of cereal or other easy to digest solid with .66-.83 oz. or 4-5 teaspoons of breast milk or formula twice a day.

Feeding Chart: 6-8 Months

BREASTMILK	AMOUNT: As frequently as baby demands (at least every 3–4 hours), along with solids
FORMULA	AMOUNT: Up to 37 oz per day, with solids INTAKE RANGE: 24–37 oz per day ## Quick Tips Give your baby a bit of formula before feeding her the solid food, to take the edge off her hunger. Once she finishes the solids, try giving her a bit more formula to see if she is still hungry. Give a full bottle (8 oz) before putting her to bed.
SOLIDS Cereals & Grains	AMOUNT: .5-2.5 oz or 1–5 tablespoons mixed with formula per day ## Quick Tips When starting baby on cereals, feed one type of grain at a time to make sure there are no allergic reactions. If your baby takes them well, you can try mixing them together for variety of taste and nutrients. OPTIONS: Rice, barley, oats
Fruits	AMOUNT: 2-4 oz or 4–8 tablespoons per day ## Quick Tips Begin making your own fruit combinations once baby has had several fruits without any allergic reaction(s). OPTIONS: Avocado, apples, bananas, apricots, mangos, nectarines, peaches, pears, plums, prunes, pumpkin

Feeding Chart: 6-8 Months, con't.

Vegetables	AMOUNT: 2-4 oz or 4–8 tablespoons per day **Quick Tips** Time for some veggie combos. Make sure your baby has tried all the vegetables first, and had no reactions prior to mixing & matching. If your baby doesn't like something at first, give it a few tries. Babies' tastes change as they mature. OPTIONS: Sweet potatoes, acorn/butternut squash, carrots, green beans, peas, yellow squash/zucchini, parsnips
Protein	AMOUNT: 1-2 oz or 2–4 tablespoons per day **Quick Tips** Try offering tofu finger cubes dusted with cereal "dust" (helps baby grasp slippery foods). Many pediatricians now recommend meats as first foods, due to the iron content. OPTIONS: Turkey, chicken, tofu
Dairy	AMOUNT: 1–2 oz or 2–4 tablespoons per day **Quick Tips** Babies love yogurt and mild cheeses. Mix yogurt with a favorite fruit puree for a breakfast treat.

Feeding Chart: 8-10 Months

BREASTMILK	AMOUNT: As frequently as baby demands (at least every 4-5 hours), along with solids
FORMULA	AMOUNT: Up to 31 oz per day with solids INTAKE RANGE: 24–31 oz per day
SOLIDS Cereals & Grains	AMOUNT: 1.5–2.5 oz or 3–5 tablespoons mixed with formula per day **Quick Tips** • Begin offering breads and muffins when baby has mastered mashed and more textured foods. • Pasta makes a great finger food. OPTIONS: Flax, graham crackers, kamut, quinoa, millet, multi-grain, crackers, whole grain Cheerios, wheat & wheat germ, toast
Fruits	AMOUNT: 2-4 oz or 4–8 tablespoons per day **Quick Tips** • Try offering raw, ripe fruits. • Soft-cooked fruits make great finger foods. OPTIONS: Blueberries, cantaloupe & melons, cherries, cranberries, dates, figs, grapes (peeled and mashed into other foods only), kiwi, papaya

Feeding Chart: 8-10 Months, con't.

Vegetables	AMOUNT: 2-4 oz or 4–8 tablespoons per day **Quick Tips** • Soft-cooked veggies make great finger foods. • Try mixing up a veggie medley. Add grated cheese for extra yum. • Sauté or roast onions or peppers to add to baby's food, or serve as finger foods. OPTIONS: Asparagus, broccoli, cauliflower, eggplant, white potatoes, onions, peppers, leeks, mushrooms, parsnips
Protein	AMOUNT: 1-2 oz or 2–4 tablespoons per day **Quick Tips** • Continue to offer a variety of foods. An omelet is the perfect chance to slip in some veggies. OPTIONS: Eggs, beans/legumes, beef, chicken, pork, ham, fish
Dairy	AMOUNT: 2-3 oz or 4–6 tablespoons per day **Quick Tips** • Get adventurous with cheeses and yogurts. Avocado mashed with a bit of cream cheese. Mmm! OPTIONS: Cream cheese, cottage cheese, colby jack, cheddars

Feeding Chart: 10-12 Months

BREASTMILK	AMOUNT: As frequently as baby demands (at least every 4-5 hours), along with solids
FORMULA	AMOUNT: Up to 31 oz per day with solids INTAKE RANGE: 24–31 oz per day
SOLIDS Cereals & Grains	AMOUNT: 2.5–4 oz or 5-8 tablespoons mixed with formula per day **Quick Tips** Break out the shaped pasta. Create your own baby pasta salad with favorite veggies and cheeses. OPTIONS: Pastas, wheat cereals, bagels
Fruits	AMOUNT: 2-4 oz or 4–8 tablespoons per day **Quick Tips** Go slowly if introducing citrus fruits. Watch for possible reactions to acidity. OPTIONS: Berries, cherries, citrus, dates, grapes (cut in quarters to avoid choking hazard)
Vegetables	AMOUNT: 2-4 oz or 4–8 tablespoons per day **Quick Tips** Try mixing up a soft-cooked, diced veggie medley. Slowly introduce tomato and other acidic foods. Watch for reactions to the acidity. OPTIONS: Artichokes, beets, corn, cucumbers, spinach, tomatoes

Feeding Chart: 10-12 Months, con't.

Protein	AMOUNT: 1-2 oz or 2–4 tablespoons per day **Quick Tips** My babies love baked fish plain or breaded. Offer with steamed veggies for a healthy meal.
Dairy	AMOUNT FOR 10-12 MONTHS OLD: 3 oz or 6 tablespoons per day AMOUNT FOR 12 MONTHS OR OLDER: 16–24 oz per day OPTIONS: Whole milk as a drink, stronger cheddars, gouda, munster, provolone, swiss, feta, brie
Sweeteners	When baby is 12 months, you can introduce raw honey

Sources: American Academy of Pediatrics, Pump Station, Sanford Health, Wholesome Babyfood.com

Vaccination Schedule: 0-6 Years

from the American Academy of Pediatrics

0-6 Years				
2 Months	Pentacel	Hepatitis B	Prevnar	Rotateq
4 Months	Pentacel	Hepatitis B	Prevnar	Rotateq
6 Months	Pentacel	Hepatitis B	Prevnar	Rotateq
10 Months	Check Hemoglobin and lead levels			
12 Months	MMR	Prevnar	Hepatitis A	TB skin test
15 Months	DTaP	HIB	Varicella	
18 Months	Hepatitis A			
2 Years	Lead Level			
3 Years	TB skin test			
4 Years	MMR	Varicella	Check Hemoglobin/ Cholesterol	
5 Years	DTaP	POLIO	TB skin test	
11 Years	TdaP	HPV	Menactra	
TB skin test annually after age 5				

DTap: Diptheria, Tetanus, Pertussis (whooping cough)
HIB: Haemophilus Influenzae Type B (meningitis)
HPV: Human Papilloma Vaccine (cervical cancer)
Menactra: Meningitis
MMR: Measles, Mumps, Rubella
Pentacel: Diptheria, Tetanus, Pertussis (whooping cough), Polio, HIB
Prevnar: Pneumococcal Bacteria (Pneumonia, Meningitis)
Rotateq: Rotavirus (diarrhea)
TdaP: Tetanus, Diptheria, Pertussis (whooping cough) Booster
Varicella: Chicken Pox

American Academy of Pediatrics: www.aap.org
Center for Disease Control and Prevention: www.cdc.gov
American Medical Association: www.ama-assn.org
National Network for Immunization Information: www.immunizationinfo.org

Notes

CHAPTER 3

p.11   ...*caloric increase during pregnancy...* "Pregnancy weight gain: What's healthy?" Mayo Clinic. www.mayoclinic.com/health/pregnancy-weight-gain/PR00111.

p.12   ... *pregnancy weight gain* ... "Weight Gain During Pregnancy Resource Sheet, table 1." Institute of Medicine 2009. www.iom.edu.

p.13   ...*essential nutrients...* "Pregnancy diet: Focus on these essential nutrients." Mayo Clinic. www.mayoclinic.com/health/pregnancy-nutrition/PR00110.

p.14   ...*iodine pregnancy dosage...* "Iodine Quick Facts." National Institute of Health. http://ods.od.nih.gov/factsheets/Iodine-QuickFacts.

p.15   ...*chocolate fats...* "Heart-Health Benefits of Chocolate Unveiled." Cleveland Clinic. http://my.clevelandclinic.org.

p.16   ...*healthy fats...* "Nutrition for Everyone. Polyunsaturated Fats and Monounsaturated Fats." Centers for Disease Control and Prevention. www.cdc.gov.

p.17   ...*recommended sugar intake...* "Sugars and Carbohydrates." American Heart Association June, 2012. www.heart.org.

p.17   …*antioxidants in sweeteners*… Phillips, Katherine M., Carlsen, Monica H., and Blomhoff, Rune. "Total Antioxidant Content of Alternatives to Refined Sugar." *Journal of the American Dietetic Association* 2009:109:64-71.

p.17   …*artificial sweeteners*… Eglash, Joanne. "Holistic Physician Dr. Andrew Weil Explains His 7 Steps to Your Perfect Weight." *Examiner* 1 May, 2012. www.examiner.com.

p.18   …*fish and mercury*… EPA-FDA Joint Federal Advisory for Mercury in Fish: "What you need to know about mercury in fish and shellfish." Environmental Protection Agency, updated 7 February, 2012. www.epa.gov/hg/advisories.htm.

p.18-9 … *foods to avoid*… Safe Eats. Food and Drug Administration. www.fda.gov.

p.19   … *pesticides and pregnancy*… Peeples, Lynn. "Dangers Posed by Pesticides During Pregnancy." *The Huffington Post* 5 April, 2012. www.huffingtonpost.com.

p.19   … *buying organics*… "When buying organic pays (and doesn't)." *Consumer Reports* June 2008. http://news.consumerreports.org.

p.20   …*pesticides in produce*… "EWG's 2012 Shopper's Guide to Pesticides in Produce™." Environmental Working Group 2012. www.ewg.org/foodnews/summary.

CHAPTER 4

p.27   …*prenatal vitamins*… "Prenatal vitamins: Why they matter, how to choose." Mayo Clinic. www.mayoclinic.com/health/prenatal-vitamins/PR00160.

p.28   …*iodine dosage*… "Iodine Quick Facts." National Institute of Health, reviewed 24 June, 2011. http://ods.od.nih.gov/factsheets/Iodine-QuickFacts.

p.29   …*chromium in water*… Layton, Lyndsey. "Probable Carcinogen Hexavalent Chromium Found in Drinking Water of 31 U.S. Cities." *The Washington Post* 19 December, 2010. www.washingtonpost.com.

p.29   ...*water filters*... "Get a Water Filter." Environmental Working Group. www.ewg.org/tap-water/getawaterfilter.

p.29   ...*herbal teas*... "Herbal Teas During Pregnancy." Baby Center. www.babycenter.com.

p.30   ...*exercise guidelines*... "Physical Activity Guidelines for Americans." U.S. Department of Health and Human Services 2008. www.hhs.gov.

p.31   ...*nature walks*... O'Connor, Anahad. "The Claim: Exposure to Plants and Parks Can Boost Immunity." *New York Times* 5 July, 2010. www.nytimes.com/2010/07/06/health.

CHAPTER 5

p.39   ...*stretch marks*... "Prevention." Mayo Clinic. www.mayoclinic.com/health/stretch-marks/DS01081.

CHAPTER 6

p.45   ...*mind-body connection*... Harris, Dan and Brady, Erin. "Re-Wiring Your Brain for Happiness: Research Shows How Meditation Can Physically Change the Brain." ABC News 28 July, 2011. http://abcnews.go.com.

p.46   ... *stress and pregnancy* ... McAdams, Patricia. "Mother's Stress May Affect Fetus." *The Washington Post* 26 September, 2006. www.washingtonpost.com.

p.46   ...*fetus experiences mother's moods*... Hamzelou, Jessica. "If Mum is Happy and You Know It, Wave Your Fetal Arms." *New Scientist* 16 March, 2010. www.newscientist.com.

CHAPTER 7

p.49   ...*bonding in womb*... Paul, Annie Murphy (2010). *Origins: How the Nine Months Before Birth Shape the Rest of Our Lives.* New York, NY: Free Press. TED Talks lecture: "What We Learn Before We're Born." November 2011. www.ted.com.

CHAPTER 8

p.55 *...maternity leave...* Friedman, Ann. "The Maternity Leave Arms Race." *New York Magazine* 2 October, 2012. www.nymag.com.

CHAPTER 13

p.82-3 *...what do babies know?...* Hirsh-Pasek, Kathy and Golinkoff, Roberta Michnick, with Eyer, Diane (2003). *Einstein Never Used Flash Cards.* New York, NY: Rodale.

CHAPTER 15

p.99 *...pacifiers...* "Pacifiers: are they good for your baby?" Mayo Clinic. www.mayoclinic.com/health/pacifiers/PR00067.

CHAPTER 17

p.128 *... baby soothing...* Karp M.D., Harvey (2002). *The Happiest Baby on the Block: The New Way to Calm Crying and Help Your Newborn Baby Sleep Longer.* New York, NY: Bantam Books.

CHAPTER 18

p.137 *...crib safety...* "Crib Safety Tips." Document #5030. U.S. Consumer Product Safety Commission. www.cpsc.gov.

CHAPTER 19

p.141 *...vaccinations adjuvants...* Northrup M.D., Christiane (2010). *Women's Bodies, Women's Wisdom.* New York, NY: Bantam Books.

CHAPTER 21

p.154 *...vulnerability...* Brown, Brené (2010). *The Gifts of Imperfection: Let Go of Who You Think You're Supposed to Be and Embrace Who You Are.* Center City, MN: Hazelden. TED Talks lecture: "The Power of Vulnerability." December 2010. www.ted.com.

Index

CPSIA information can be obtained at www.ICGtesting.com
Printed in the USA
LVOW02s1057140414

381617LV00008B/19/P

9 780988 871205